Red
(Scarlet)
Flags
Unheeded

Ophelia Olive Reim

ISBN 978-1-0980-9519-2 (paperback)
ISBN 978-1-0980-9521-5 (hardcover)
ISBN 978-1-0980-9520-8 (digital)

Christian Faith Publishing, Inc.
832 Park Avenue
Meadville, PA 16335
www.christianfaithpublishing.com

Printed in the United States of America

Everyone who knows what is the right thing
to do, and doesn't do it, commits sin.
—James 4:17

I dedicate this evolvement of a memento to my son. As a witness to his steadfastness, his loyalty, his compassion, and his unconditional love, silently and strongly, he has compelled me to persevere, to continue attempting to be the woman God has created me to be in this earthen vessel.

In gratitude for his careful words, his unhurried visits, his endless open mind to my words and ways, his invitations to listen to what I feel is important to share…for this and much, much more, I give God the glory, giving thanks for my son.

For all these mysteries I thank you; for the wonder of myself, for the wonder of your works.
—Psalm 139:14

Discourse

This is *my* personal accounting about a stark unplanned episode in my life, a sharing of a continual adaptation to repercussions stemming from an event which was unauthorized by me. Me, a surviving (albeit minute by minute), struggling, and traumatized victim of an attempted deliberate homicide, who most often feels as if she is hardly existing.

> Peace I bequeath to you, my own peace the world cannot give, this is my gift to you.
> —John 14:27

This is *my* journey. Me, tirelessly reliving a hideous victimization which should have been interrupted by the attentiveness toward, and a subsequent intervention of, the many screaming red (scarlet) flags that went deplorably unheeded—unheeded by so many: family, friends, classmates, teachers, administrators on various levels, law enforcement personnel, and perhaps others who daily interacted with the sixteen-year-old student who ultimately had a plan to kill me and sexually assault my corpse. These individuals who became and remained firm in their thoughts, words, actions, and their opinions regarding the inconsistencies, the many unknowns, the unanswered, the confusions and incongruencies and allowed obscurities, which were to remain status quo, were *acceptable* to all of them. This united acceptance of chaos and immorality in many areas involving many people is a detriment to society. Evilness filled the peoples.

> What I want to say is this; my sorrow is so
> great, my mental anguish so endless.
> —Romans 9:2

My days are often confusing, frequently feeling feeble, a lane laden with erratic uncertain intricacies. Confusion, stymied perhaps. My pass is not commonly traveled; it's truly not a place wherein I have the abilities to pull myself up out of the obscurity that is enveloping me. Obscurity within entities created obscurity in my existence.

It's a lane I am very unfamiliar with, a lane which oftentimes randomly shifts into an unpredictable carousal—a continual disordering with no footing.

> He robs the depths of their darkness,
> brings deep shadow to the light.
> —Job 12:22

It is now that the time feels right.

The Holy Spirit is encouraging me, gently stirring me, and I truly recognize and accept that truly this time, yes, this time, the time has arrived for me to share the truism of this astounding unchartered travel.

A manifest of unnecessary losses which is an inconclusive list by far of my losses…my laughter, my joy, and my peace, which were once exuberantly lived out, were vastly and quickly snuffed out by red (scarlet) flags unheeded.

To absolve the guilty and condemn the virtuous, both alike are abhorrent to Yahweh.
—Proverbs 17:15

Prayer is the foundation of my being and that reality encapsulates all that goes forward with every breath I breathe. Always offering others' prayer requests, I fervently make these supplications to the Lord; however, I especially now have my own aching supplications as I turn toward God for all humanity, praying he guides all to error on the side of prudence by sharing their knowledge of probable detriment they are akin to, with the *appropriate authorities (all of them, dismissing none).* Divulging of information may possibly save someone's life or may at least prevent the sorrow and trials of one struggling to even just remain in her body.

So always treat others as you would like
them to treat you; this is the meaning
of the Law and the Prophets.
—Matthew 7:12

I ask the Holy Spirit, in even the most miniscule of ways, to nudge all people, inspire them
in that holy prodding, which is oftentimes a soft,
gentle touch, to share the knowledge (with proper
authorities) that they have about a potential undiagnosed mental illness or the witnessing of disconcerting and strange behaviors or abnormal activities, especially and not excluding *knowledge of the
fantasies of a failing high school student to carry out
a hideous crime,* among many other disconcerting
fantasies, to gain pleasure.

More than all else, keep watch over your
heart, since here are the wellsprings of life.
—Proverbs 4:23

Holding on to secrets, omitting information,
ostensibly investigating, and deliberately ignoring
and making a great effort to avoid what you see or
hear is wrong and unjust and your inaction can and
oftentimes will cause irreparable damage—damages to a body, mind, soul, and spirit, most likely
not your own, notably at this present time. If you
haven't been subject to others' (a lot of others, in
some cases) lack of conscience and the adamant

dismissal of sharing dangerous truths, know that secrets do advance to maiming and killing. If you are at all a conscionable human being, if even at the slightest of degrees on the continuum of breathing, and you maintain mental health or even just the rudimentary knowledge of what is right and what is wrong, you have a moral obligation toward humanity to put others' welfare ahead (could be your own welfare in jeopardy) of your delights, your goals, your dreams and self-imposed "loving your earthly life" conveniences of "not wanting to get involved," detriment of jeopardizing the climbing a ladder of a prized success, possibly sabotaging your financial wealth, fears of the loss of your relationships, promises to keep silent, adhering to the contracts which were signed, protecting one another's status, agreed upon loyalty to a friend or lover, remaining in a favorite circle. Put simply, living out a loyalty (no matter what the cost is to others) to an idol that you make a choice to bow down to while jeopardizing life and limb of another is sinful.

Trouble is coming to the man who grossly exploits others for the sake of his house, to fix his nest on high and so evade the hand of misfortune.
—Habakkuk 2:9

Loyalty to idols is costly, oftentimes to the death of another's known existence.

Because the teraphim utter futile words and
the diviners have lying visions and publish
empty dreams and voice misleading nonsense,
naturally the people stray like sheep; they
wander because they have no shepherd.
—Zechariah 10:2

It sounds quite elementary, but be honest and have self-respect and in turn, respect for *all* humanity, *whether or not* you are entitled to an *immunity* within the position you hold (whereby, you will likely be exonerated, whether you tell the truth *or* withhold the truth) *or not*. Immunity must be granted to the righteous, sans those who chose immorality.

Having nothing to do with the futile works
of darkness but exposing them by contrast.
—Ephesians 5:11

Do not be embarrassed in not following "the" crowd or acting arrogantly, but shout out your truths even though it may be independent of your in-group's choices or a judge's ruling that a tragedy in her eyes was "unforeseeable." The lack of honesty and the subsequent injustices and the inactions that occurred in so many opportunistic interventions over a period of years is egregious. Unfortunately, the decisions made by many individuals to withhold information and ultimately to withhold the truth, in unity with a reprehensible lack of thoroughness in determining accountability, have caused annihilation, disfigurement, crippling, pain, and suffering in many different ways.

You must not love this passing world or anything that is in the world. The love of the Father cannot be in any man who loves the world, because nothing the world has to offer—the sensual body, the lustful eye, pride in possessions—could ever come from the Father but only from the world, with all it craves for, is coming to an end; but anyone who does the will of God remains forever.
—1 John 2:15–17

Leadership and administration consisting of a principal, numerous assistant principals, various counselors, many educators (even reportedly), a student resource officer from the local police department, in addition to many other individuals in the community such as parents, classmates, and friends, had the knowledge of a troubled teenage boy, and all had the ability and the responsibility to thwart a disturbing, violent tragedy, whose infamous origination *began with* the writing assignment of a sophomore high school student, participating in a common, accredited high school classroom, in the United States of America, in Montana, on January, 7, 2002.

Do not let anyone deceive you with empty arguments; it is for this loose living that God's anger comes down on those who rebel against him. Make sure that you are not included with them. You were darkness once, but now you are light in the Lord; be like children of light, for the effects of the light are seen in complete goodness and right living and truth. Try to discover what the Lord wants of you, having nothing to do with the futile works of darkness but exposing them by contrast. The things which are done in secret are things that people are ashamed even to speak of; but anything exposed by the light will be illuminated, and anything illuminated turns into light. That is why it is said: Wake up from your sleep, rise from the dead, and Christ will shine on you.

—Ephesians 5:6–14

High school assignment is titled and turned in to the assigning teacher as

"Comp New Year's Resolution
1/7/2002, 11:19 a.m."

(assignment was turned over to
administration / school leadership / supervisors
ten days later, on January 17, 2002)

For there is nothing hidden but it must
be disclosed, nothing kept secret except
to be brought to light. If anyone has
ears to hear, let him listen to this.
—Mark 4:22–23

Each day, wakefulness becomes confusing, often crippling and toilsome. Nighttime is a weary place and an expected eerie, nightmare-filled place. I try to smile as I continually attempt to live in a sought-after serenity, a calmness above this calamitous base of the liabilities acquired by the preventable devastation which has resulted in traumatic brain injury, post-traumatic stress disorder (which in and of itself is comprised of many ailments), anxiety, depression, chronic pain, arthritis and, sadly as I write in tears, a degeneration of my being.

Obscurity led to a betrayal surrounded by sufferings of more than one can grasp.

Bless those who curse you, pray for
those who treat you badly.
—Luke 6:28

The incessant aggressive ills bring
assaults upon me with every breath I take.
Isolation; loss of friendships; short-term memory
issues; agitation; fatigue; nightmares; impatience;
impulsivities; constant
medical care; physical, mental, social, and
emotional suffering; unemployment; financial
strains; hypervigilance, watchfulness; and
sorrows…this condensed list of maladies
is an encapsulation of what veritably
remains of me. My world is complicated.
The persistent infirmities
constrain me to occupy my own island—a
foreigner in my shell, in a world
of one.

I stay awake, lamenting like a
lone bird on the roof.
—Psalm 102:7

Years beyond the tragedy (my victim statement to the offender)

Today is the day you will leave the confines of your prison stay. I hold no grudge, Dick. I am sincere when I tell you that I have no disdain toward you. It is my hope for you that you experience a productive, peaceful life. I forgave you years ago. Actually I never felt I had hardened my heart toward you, ever. I was never hateful toward you. I was concerned about you. I hope that you in some way felt loved and cared about while you were serving your prison sentence as you truly were only a child. I hope you had someone to talk to, someone to lean on. In my heart, I know those who were obligated to raise you with love, attention, and charged to guard you...failed you. In addition to your family and friends, the school system allowed you to fail in the school setting, but not solely in academics. You must have felt that no one cared. You must have felt that you had no one to turn to, to look up to, to protect you. It appears you had no one to hear you, no one to truly listen to you. That saddens me. You were failed by those who were obligated to protect you and help you grow healthfully in mind, body, soul, and spirit. I feel bad that you were ignored and abandoned. If I had known you then, I would have done all I could have to help you navigate to the necessities of a healthy life.

Not a day goes by that I don't think about what you did to me on Tuesday, May 27, 2003, at dusk. Remember that early evening? It was a gorgeous evening, just after suppertime, and my son and I recently returned home from a two-mile walk and jog to the middle school. We ran into my coworker and friend who also was out and about. We talked and laughed for a few minutes and reminded each other we would see each other the next day at work. Well, we thought we would see each other the next day at work… Unfortunately, we were wrong.

I don't know if you know this or not. I'm not sure what you knew about me actually. I had a position in the school district that I loved! I was relied upon to help elementary school children progress in their reading skills and advance in their mathematical skills. I was the assigned individual to tutor them one-on-one, and I loved where I was at. Your decision to strike me with your massive Dodge Ram, revving thirty miles an hour up over the curb and onto the sidewalk where I was walking and jogging, ended that brand-new career. Of course, that's not the only area of my life your choices adversely affected, but I mention that because education is something I hold dear to my heart and helping those who were struggling was my own private mission. I took great pride in helping those who sometimes needed an extra few minutes of attention in their studies.

My back aches, my neck extremely fatigued, constantly rearranging my position (my entire body and my neck) as I sit down to write this letter to you; the writing of facts of how your decision to strike me *impacts* my moment to moment survival. Survive—yes, that's what I do, Dick, survive. Did you notice how I got off track from the lines up above? When you struck me from behind at my hips, my body fell backward onto the hood of your Ram truck then whiplashed again forward as you continued on, dragging my lifeless body underneath your truck for twenty-five feet until my body somehow finally lost the connection to the metal attachments on your truck. My forehead forcefully hit the pavement and your decision to follow through with your *number 1* New Year's Resolution (get a driver's license so I can do those horrible things people like to read about in the paper) was deemed by you a success (by me, a partial success). Your friend in the passenger seat told the police that you were excited to accomplish this feat. I guess some people would call this a success of a resolution; I call it a sin-filled crime. I am not going to mince words. You've had enough misdirection and falsities in your life shown and verbalized to you by a lot of people in all walks of life for so many years, and I refuse to contribute to their waywardness and misguidances. I am straight with you, and I will be honest.

Well, I say "partial" success because when you came back to retrieve my body after taking Pat, your friend of eight years, home, and to finish what it was you wanted to do with my body (body to me, your hope was for a corpse), some first responders had just arrived to take me to the hospital. The police reports denote that students at your high school across the street from where you dragged me heard me screaming in terror and the residents whose house I just jogged by saw me out their windows and then witnessed you driving your truck up onto the sidewalk aiming straight at me. This is all hearsay to me. I wasn't cognizant after the strike. Angels were among me though. Unbeknownst to me, those residents selflessly covered me with a homemade quilt and the students from your high school stayed with me to give me comfort until the first responders arrived. I have no clue that they comforted me or not; that's just what I heard and have read. These people rescued me before you returned to pick up my body and sexually assault me. Physically, I was somewhat saved. Being informed of the picture you had inside the truck console, I cringe. Remember the picture of the burning woman in your truck that was found as evidence? To this day the imagination of that picture makes me shudder. I get sick to my stomach envisioning you burning my body. Many years later, I still shake my head in disbelief. Had we met before? Had I shown you disrespect prior to this meeting that enticed you to attempt to take away my life and use my corpse for ill?

Not surprisingly, my son and his father heard the sirens (we lived about eight blocks away from the attempted deliberate homicide scene) as law enforcement officers and the fire department personnel were dispatched to the crime scene.

My heart aches for my son every day. As I was unable to communicate at all, straddling consciousness and unconsciousness, the chaplain at the hospital would not be able to hold off the truth any longer and was forced to inform my son that "your mom may not make it." I cry to this day, envisioning my son in the emergency room halls, but in a room away from my lifeless body, listening to and looking into the eyes of a man of God he had never met, tell him that regardless of the upcoming days, our lives were forever changed. Indeed, forever changed and magnanimously concerning.

You turned our lives into something unimaginable. You turned my family upside down and sideways and the aftermath of it all is indescribable in all ways possible, always a surprise of random demises.

You played dirty with my family, and you didn't think (maybe, you didn't even care) how this would affect me and those dear to me. It's probable you didn't know I had a fourteen-year-old son who would soon be graduating from middle school, *truly, at the end of that week*! Maybe you did know. Maybe you knew more about me and my family than you divulged to your passenger Pat and to the police officers. Maybe you have seen my son and I enjoying the evenings together all spring-time long. Your family and our family do live quite near to one another; anything is possible. Maybe you knew more about us than I thought you knew, or you led everyone on to believe you knew. There are many unknowns. So very many questions have remained unanswered. This crime and the information regarding the events during the months and the years leading up to this specific tragedy are filled with inconsistencies, obscurities, inconclusiveness, and confusion. I have learned just what "fatty chaos" is truly all about.

I recently had helped my son's teachers prepare for the eighth-grade students' graduation; unfortunately I was a victim of a tragedy and unable to participate in life's events whatsoever, including attending my son's graduation ceremony because I was hospitalized. I was just being moved out of the intensive care unit to another floor the moment he was graduating. To this day, I cry. My son grew up rather quickly in so many of the moments and days of continual heartache and disbelief. Stolen, his innocence and childlike joy, stolen. That twinkle in his eye…

Back to the lines I had written way up above… You see, when you dragged me, the frontal lobe of my brain was severely injured. Those cells were killed. Your violent feat left me with a traumatic brain injury. The repercussions of this have left me to be a person I was not. On that beautiful evening you ran me over and dragged me, hoping to see my death and subsequently participate in a fantasy of a sexual assault. You depleted much of my being, but not only my being.

When you struck me with your truck, you hit me so hard and fast that when my forehead hit the ground, my brain ricocheted from back to front. But the initial hit before being dragged, it was then that my brain ricocheted from front to back. Pat, your passenger and friend, told the police officers investigating this crime that you were going about thirty miles per hour. It's unfortunate you didn't get a flat tire jumping that curb to interrupt your fantasy. Too bad Pat didn't in some way try to interrupt the completion of this crime. He could have yelled out to me, or instead of watching your attempts to kill me, he could have turned the steering wheel. Of course he probably thought then that he would get hurt or killed. He was just as criminal-acting as you were, Dick. It sounds like you were determined to accomplish this no matter what, so a flat tire wasn't going to stop you. You had made up your mind over four hundred days earlier that you were going to commit this crime, eventually.

These years since the attack have been very difficult for me and also for those near to me. Your premeditated criminal act has impaired me in many ways physically, emotionally, mentally, socially, and yes, spiritually.

Because of your decision to follow through with your number one resolution on your Composition New Year's Resolution assignment, I now have a very debilitating short-term memory issue, united with a traumatic brain injury, which contributes to difficulty concentrating, agitation, impulsivity, impatience, perpetual distractions, and irritability. This may sound like an elementary feat to you, but I can't place documents in date or numerical order in a timely fashion as I once accomplished, and I am now perpetually distracted from the time I get up until the day's end. I am now someone who I don't know. If I leave something I began, even only to turn my head, the chore I began no longer exists. A physician in the area evaluated me after the incident and he calls that characteristic "out of sight, out of mind." The brain injury is a constant reminder of you. I cannot accomplish what I once was very confident in completing. I am saddened, humiliated, and frustrated. These ailments I endure are excessive in number and can be very dangerous at times. It's amazing the house hasn't burned down, nor the house becoming flooded. It's surprising that not all my clothing is damaged and unwearable. Yeah, it's pretty unbelievable how a person can be changed in truly just a couple of minutes (underneath your truck). Chaos demands my attention.

This me is unfamiliar to myself and to others. My demise is what you say made you feel exhilarated and powerful. Sounds like my detriment was your awesomeness.

You literally stole so much of my once-healthy brain. Noises, movements, light (anything my senses respond to) smells and fragrances sicken me. I am startled always and respond in fear to most things. Everything is a threat to me. You, once a complete stranger, have become a part of my everyday existence; however, I do not know you. I just know "of" you.

When people try to get my attention, they aren't trying to startle me; they just don't realize that I am on guard every waking moment. They don't mean any harm to me, but being approached by them, they see and feel the fear of my response; they cannot predict my response nor calm the screams of terror. My days are filled with tears and fears.

You have scarred me, and I wonder which one of my startled responses will stop my beating heart, having kept beating now for so long through startling responses and always unknowingly threatened by the next innocent interaction. I wonder if my heart will soon have had enough of enduring the trauma (like my emotions have); the perpetual startled-response existence many times a day which keep the flow of chemicals on an ongoing high alert and operating in confusion. It's very fatiguing, it's very lonely, and often feel I am succumbing to a very sorrowful existence.

The providers' diagnoses of PTSD, major depression, and generalized anxiety disorder, in addition to the TBI and the extensive number of symptoms, have evolved into a difficult existence for myself. United with those everlasting disabilities are chronic body and nerve pain and mobilization loss from all the fractures I sustained as I was struck and dragged for twenty-five feet. There have been many times in the past years that I have wished that you would have fully succeeded in your quest and ultimately killed me. This new and challenging way of functioning is very confusing, costly, and draining in many ways; the burdens financially are impressive; the demise of relationships and an inability to sustain them are ongoing and very isolating, an extremely lonely survival. I am alone. You may understand how hard it is to trust anyone; home is where I stay. This is where I feel safe, in my room. These ailments affect all parts of my being and the oftentimes chaotic management of my daily life. Continually irritated and annoyed with noises, loudness, the inability to concentrate and always distracted, it's a confusing existence adding in a short-term memory issue and other effects on the frontal lobe of my brain. Much of me has been manipulated without my authorization, much has been lost. What I see and often feel is a puzzled shell—a puzzled shell laden in fear and tears.

You were excited to get your driver's license.

I have difficulty driving. Riding as a passenger isn't hardly enjoyable either anymore. "Makes sense though," I think to myself. I don't want to hear the loud noise of a vehicle behind me; I can't use my rearview mirror as there is so much anxiety having anyone behind me. They drive too closely to me! They frighten me! It is not enjoyable for me to take a walk. Sometimes people don't stay on the road when they are driving, and even as I follow city ordinances to walk on the sidewalks and not on the public streets and roadways, I can still get hit. Anything is possible.

When you and I met, well, when we clashed, I used to walk two to six miles to exercise. Today? Much has changed in my life. It's very difficult to exercise when the entire body aches and managing all the other disabilities, with overall balance for the moment, being the goal. Physical therapy was fruitful but they do not let patients continue treatment if there is not anything they can further do to assist one with chronic pains and immobility. I am learning to accept constant pain. I was discharged from physical therapy. I have to figure out much on my own. I'm not sure if you are aware of the damages to my body. In case you didn't read the local or the national newspapers, I will share with you why I have the sorrow, fears, exaggerated emotions and pains, and much more debilitation. Besides the traumatic brain injury (which alone encapsulates tens of ailments), my spinal processes on each side of my spine were fractured, I sustained broken ribs and a punctured lung, severe whiplash with continual problems in my neck and shoulders, nose fractures and affected sinuses, four pelvic fractures, and a tailbone fracture. My teeth were a sight of brokenness; the cement was very hard, and at thirty miles per hour, parts of my flesh and teeth remain embedded on that alleyway across from your school. From my head to my toes, I was a package of concrete and sand-filled wounds. For nearly a month I was hospitalized in ICU, recovery, and rehabilitation. I don't remember being there, but I suffered much, and now I continue to try to placate the constant pain. Naturally, I feel broken with wrenching pains. The lump on my forehead which signifies the frontal lobe of my brain greets me every time I look into the mirror. I see you every day when I wake up. I feel every pain and think of you before bed.

The completion of your number 1 resolution on your New Year's Resolution assignment does not let me forget, even for one moment, how you have taken away so much of the "used to be me." You are literally in my face every new day.

I often think about the evening you found me. Being the extrovert I was at that time in my life, I often wonder if I waved to you and your passenger as you two "cruised" around the area (as you scoped out which block you would choose to actually run me down on). I used to be a very friendly, outgoing, bubbly, joyful woman up until May 27, 2003, 8:46 p.m., my fortieth year of this life. I don't trust others, and I question others' laughter and frivolity. I wonder why a lot of people are so happy, smiling, and joking. Your decision has left me a miserable, confused, and hurting shell. The best time of my day is at 7:00 p.m. That's when I will try to go to bed and try to forget how miserable I am and try to get away from the pains of many sorts.

Prior to the impact, during the acceleration to get up over the curb, did you wonder if I had responsibilities in my life, such as being a competent loving parent to a child? Perhaps you did see me with my son twenty minutes earlier a couple of miles away from where you struck me. I was nearer your home twenty minutes earlier, so maybe you did see us joking, smiling, and laughing. From your house to the middle school is likely a few minutes, then from the middle school to our house is about ten minutes. Yeah, it's quite possible we all crossed paths just moments before the incident. I can't say for sure, but perhaps you were scouting out my demise a little earlier in the evening, even earlier than law enforcement had believed and had reported. There's not a whole lot in the police reports I've read time and time again… So many unanswered questions. You took my son's childhood away from him. After you did your damage to me, my son did all he could to help me in recovery;

yes, he helped dress me, helped me move my legs (I was a torn-up, broken mess), and he was there for me and I needed him to be with me. Thank you for not running us both down. I am grateful. My son gave me great hope to work at healing; my son had become my parent, my help. The twinkle in his eye is faint. Your actions make me cry to this day.

I am mad, sad, and disappointed about much (but certainly forgiving, as I said earlier) that you and your passenger didn't stop to think about many things before you ran me down. I look back again and again and am thankful my son was through trick riding for the day when I iterated to him that I wanted to spend just a little bit more time outside in the springtime weather. I wanted to walk and maybe jog a little bit more. I placed eight quarters into my pocket, and off I trotted to Albertson's (well, that was the plan anyway). I was going to surprise my upcoming graduate with a couple of candy bars; he was graduating in three days from middle school, and I just thought it would be a fun gesture to treat him in even just a small way even though he never had much of a sweet tooth! I wanted to make these last few days before middle-school graduation exciting, fun, and memorable... Oh, they would be memorable all right.

Evidence at the crime scene: two quarters, a hair clip, and blood. I never did get my tennis shoes back from the evidence room at the police department. I suppose there was too much blood on them. I don't know what attachment it was on your truck, but that rusty attachment sliced deeply into my left side sliding downward into my left hip; the remnant tissue that is remaining is numb and an unrehabilitatable, sad-looking part of flesh—a large fatty permanent hematoma. A large part of my left leg has no feeling; apparently that indicates that some nerve damage was done. I had so many concerns about that tube placed into my side, watching it for days as it continually filled up with blood and other bodily fluids, always hoping that in the morning I would wake up and see that the drainage was clear and much less in volume. It took weeks to get to the point of my hopes realized. The fears of infection were always disconcerting. I had an amazing physician and assistant who checked in on me regularly, committed to their positions in health care. I prayed much to our Lord for healing, for healing in so many ways. A spiritual director gifted me with a prayer for healing. I continue to pray that written prayer each morning. The vaginal slicing was also the site of much injury and blood loss, so I agree it is not a surprise why my jogging outfit and shoes were not returned to me. I liked that outfit, my favorite colors of olive green and black.

"Exposure therapy" was unsuccessful; remaining in the house eight blocks away from the crime scene and having so many reminders of that hideous tragedy was affecting my well-being, literally compounding all the disabilities I was trying to manage physically, emotionally, socially, spiritually, and mentally. I searched for healing. I received misdirection and little guidance in the healing I so yearned for; I needed to make some big changes. It was a matter of peace. I must move out of that house and out of that part of the USA. Exposure therapy in this particular event was not fruitful; it was contributing to a demise of existence of a life that once yearned to actually live.

I made some very large changes, and I continue to search for healing. It is fleeting, but it's my job every day. My peace is dependent upon my focus to heal and manage my disabilities better than the moment before. The rest of my life, my job each breath will be to focus on healing in some way, managing the numbers of ailments as well as I can for that moment in time and continue to pray before I go to bed to be free of a nightmare, just for this night, at least, dear God!

Dispatchers in law enforcement communications offices and police officers aren't thrilled receiving 911 calls from me as I try to iterate to them I am dying, only to gradually become aware that I am breathing. I must not be dying, and they can cancel the ambulance. The police have shown up and checked my house; they logically thought maybe I was a victim of a crime. They searched my house and found no one of course. Calling the police department the following day to apologize to a sergeant that was a first responder on our particular crime scene was not easy. These unpredictable occurrences aren't experienced daily, but going through it time and again isn't fulfilling or anything to be proud of. The police sergeant kindly accepted my apology, my tears flowing. I was embarrassed, frightened I would be held criminally responsible for something I didn't mean to do. These are things that are out of my control, and I do not like feeling like I can't manage a lot of things in my life. I hurt, I cry, I hurt, I cry... I didn't want anyone to know that the damage you have done "actually" has affected me negatively each moment and has changed me much. Hiding the hundreds of disruptions you've created is constantly daunting. For many years I was ashamed, guilty to live and display my existence with these disparities. Today, I no longer cower in embarrassment of my symptoms; trying to hide hundreds of symptoms has become impossible for me. I am an enigma, I am always misunderstood, made fun of, judged ruthlessly, and most of all, I have been alienated.

These symptoms are not likened to the flu; these symptoms were specially created by you succeeding (partially) in your number one New Year's Resolution assignment. These particular symptoms evolving from the damage you created by your evil act are a prevention to the livelihood I once thrived in, the specific goals I had made for myself, and the dreams of various things I was hoping toward.

These are just a few of the many unauthorized obstacles I face.

Please don't have a reenactment of your number 1 resolution you made in 2003. Be good to others and be kind to yourself. I am not mad at you. I am frustrated and extremely disappointed with those who were responsible to seeing that your welfare was attended to. You and I were failed by many, many so-called professionals. They were not your mentors; they watched you spiral; they watched your GPA plummet to a 0.83 with no guidance to help you to get on a successful path to see that you could finish your sophomore year. Their lack of any sort of intervention, evaluation, or an assessment is unacceptable. They didn't have your success as a goal. They ignored you, and by ignoring you as if you were invisible, you felt invisible, and your road to perdition hastened. Those so-called professionals had a duty to attend to you and help you. You were crying out for help in so many ways, and everyone that had contact with you failed you. Your cries were deliberately ignored. That's heart-wrenching to me. Your loud cries over a period of years were verbal, physical, emotional, spiritual, mental, and social. I am sorry that in the hundreds of people you came into contact with on a daily basis, no one considered you worthy to be shown charity and love. No one was interested in seeking your welfare, in your obviously loud, troubled state. That is a human error. This crime was not totally your fault. Others left you to spiral into a deep dark place. They didn't consider you valuable, so by their lack of actions, they contributed to your demise. People in authority, people who were in charge of mentoring you, people paid to educate you, people who were gifted by God to have you as a son, people who monitored you academically, people who watched you throughout your school day—the list of spectators (only) is seemingly endless to me; there is no excuse for anyone to have not stepped up to help you.

God will take care of you. Believe in him who created you to be a great man, a good friend, a hard worker. God wants the best for you and so do I. Surround yourself with those who love and serve God, be gentle with yourself and be kind to yourself. It's time now for you to feel loved and cared about.

God bless you,
Ophelia

Now you must repent and turn to God,
so that your sins may be wiped out.
—Acts 3:19

In just three days, he was scheduled to become an eighth-grade graduate from middle school in a city in the center of Montana. It would most certainly be a time of many celebrations, good cheer, smiles, tears, laughter, and so much satisfaction. The hugging and the celebrating would, of course, go on for the weekend and deep into the summer months!

Involved parents meticulously prepared special events, helped construct student art profiles that would ultimately line the gymnasium where the graduation ceremony would be held, and all of us who prepared for the most amazing graduation parties across the city were certainly not only proud of their student but happy to be an integral part to create many lasting memories.

Each student arrived swiftly with excitement bursting at the seams as they entered their art classroom. Together we would embark on the final eighth-grade project in this particular classroom. Myself and another volunteer oversaw the operation of the projector and the subsequent completed amazing profiles of the bustling students, which soon would be proudly displayed on the walls where the graduation celebration would take place in only three days! It was quite clear to me after many years of spending time with these students and knowing their families that these eighth graders were assuredly securely molded and educated with great care, and now it was time to celebrate! Their kindnesses exchanged was a beautiful reminder of their well-being, and their respect and gratitude they showed to those of us volunteering to make their upcoming graduation gathering a memorable event were deeply felt. We smiled as we outlined their maturing faces, tracing with welcomed interruptions, as they moved unintentionally while beaming ear to ear, certainly indicative of the knowledge that very soon, they were to commemorate together and run toward their high school years.

The students' graduation boards which were assigned as a final project were eagerly being filled up with many heartfelt moments shared with the closely intertwined group of soon-to-be graduates. Pictures, quotes, drawings, and symbols, each board became a summary of the most memorable of times, signifying what was most important to each student in the many years they had spent together. Some entries were duplicated on one another's boards, indicating with no doubt that they truly lived some very close bonds which were becoming more and more evident as the project progressed. As each student was welcomed into the lives of their friends' families, they grew to become one family. God's family. Clearly, the working on these special boards became times of delight.

The undeniable gratitude for the students' daily experiences in the past three years was a tribute to a togetherness that none could conceal. The hours were filled with memorializing, kidding, contagious laughter, and possibly poking fun at some things, but at times, some moments were silent. In realizing that not all memories could be adhered to their boards, the students recounted their years and became acutely aware that yes, they were abundantly blessed with amazing educators, support staff, principal, and a wise patient priest who was pleased to shepherd them. It became very clear that some of the moments would never be able to be accurately conveyed. The quick-approaching Friday evening graduation would be magnanimous for many. A formal Mass and tandem celebratory service would be the perfect beginning to a ceremony that would commemorate the many eighth graders that would be deservedly graduating.

There was a silent joy in the air, so many innate proud grins of satisfaction and accomplishments as the projects were carefully and quietly completed; however, I am not certain, I really am unable to say for sure, but I typically trust my intuition, and this time I trust it greatly as I am in the students' presence and my heart is speaking quietly to me in saying, "Yes, indeed, there were some tears…"

My fortune in being a part of the completion of the students' final project will not be forgotten, nor will I take these precious times for granted. The students' undeniable gratitude for their daily experiences, lessons, growth, and surroundings, which were filled with love in this school, could not ever again be concealed.

They were being reminded of much and were taking in deeply so much during this last project; many grateful and quiet appreciative moments became common during this time. Taking time from shooting hoops and trick riding, great truths began to take hold of these students' embracing the strong feelings and vivid thoughts that they had truly received many blessings, and in the quiet ending of the assignment, their hearts were thankful.

I have iterated the students' joy, and I sincerely feel their oftentimes silent but rambunctiousness as I write about them with a smile. I also want to share that we parents who entrusted our children to the personnel at this school were very blessed and fortunate to have been active in our children's schooling as we became invitingly involved with the progress our children made as students at this very special school I will continue to hold close to my heart until my dying breath. I am so proud to have been able to be active in my child's schooling and development, and I just couldn't wait to see him beam receiving his middle-school certificate surrounded by his best friends and families. My friends and their families, this was truly going to be so special for all of us! I cannot wait!

Eager hotshot eighth graders in their favorite groups, shopping for their semiformal attire for their big night! Whirling around, making last-minute appointments for their hairstyles, highlights, and haircuts. You wonder where are the intricately involved proud parents. They are attentively smiling and shaking their heads, watching (stealthily in the background), holding tightly to the joy their children are obviously feeling. Literally palpable, the students' energy was alluring, and we were feeling and embracing our children's satisfied spirits of accomplishments. I smile... I shake my head with my own delight that, yes, I made some very good choices for my son. He has soared. He's so happy. I can see it, I can feel it, it's all so tangible... I strongly hold tight to these precious moments. I cannot wait till Friday night! This is going to be amazing!

Clearly, with their boisterous celebratory spirits ranging far and wide, the soon-to-be graduates were engrossing every minute of their last days of middle school with an unbridled exuberance. Wait. Now and then, I sense something new, perhaps a sadness in the quiet in some, it's for the most part, inaudible, but as I watch their faces, they seem to be reminded out, of nowhere, of the reality that they will be attending different high schools in the area. In the midst of the most joyful moments, these realities will remind them also of the times in which some of their former middle school classmates relocated to another city or of the times friends' parents decided to enroll them in another school in the area. This unsettling feeling becomes more familiar. They will once again be reminded of a sadness, a loss, truly a time of grieving (again). Yes, pure undeniable grief—a feeling unrecognized or perhaps undiagnosed as such, in these chapters of life in their journey, but certainly, grief. They definitely won't see one another every day, or for weeks. It's quite probable they won't even be able to make their schedules accommodate them in any way to fit in a trick bike-ride together. They may no longer shoot hoops together, they won't call on their girls together, and just as importantly, they certainly won't attend weekly school Mass together. They will all make new friends, they will embark upon a new circle—yes, this newness approaching can be very scary and an unprecedented difficult time to accept in their childhood. Some of the grins and guffaws are subsiding.

The demanding transition waits for no one! There are no "yield" signs, so certainly no "stop" signs. These unstoppable changes can and will be downright traumatizing, unexpected for some, and at the very least, surprising for all, as the once-expected familiarity and comfort will be quickly interrupted. Just like that! The routines for years of (albeit "believed") knowingness that bred security will flee. Just as all else in our existence, these former and new feelings and accompanying emotions are very real and exist as important parts of our being that must be accepted first. I can see where this sadness comes from. A sensitive soul as I am, I now feel that my heart is sad for those who are having a more difficult time with this reality. Wait! We are going to put those feelings of melancholy, anxiety, and fear aside. It's evident those are not feelings that are popular in their conversations today; besides, we must put all this aside for now as we have a celebration to attend to!

I try to move on in the much-expected jubilant, celebratory mode, but I am stuck right now. I am seriously immobile. Why at times does it seem so hard to genuinely accept and embrace whatever we are feeling at this moment? If as adults we ponder and make a plan to walk through unfamiliar, possibly wearisome times in healthful ways, imagine the confusion and difficulty a young student feels during these times when they are being expected to "figure it out," "grow up," and "get over it." That's harsh for a middle-school child to hear. That is downright immoral to rush a child through hardships, pains, and trials. Those true, raw feelings and emotions sometimes get ignored and pushed way deep down where they never will belong. It's a popular line: "Live (accept) in the moment." It's just not always possible or that easy for many to follow a popular mantra as this with so many varying issues and levels of transitions. Definitely not a helpful healthy blanket suggestion for various reasons. I must say for myself, it's quite difficult to embrace an anxiety, fresh beginnings, and share an authentic exuberance in the many unknowns that we all experience in our lives. Many things take much time to accept, embrace, plan, and exhale. My mantra has evolved to "Be soft and gentle with thyself wherever you are situated." Professed words of "wrapping our heads around something and imitating another's advice that possibly worked well for another" just isn't oftentimes realistic, healthy, nor recommended for an indefinite number of reasons. Be kind to yourself; truly care about yourself in the ways you do with those you have grown to love throughout your life. You and I deserve to be loved and cared for by our very beautiful selves, created intricately and miraculously by a loving Father.

It's commonplace to embrace unknowns with great difficultly. Living out loud, showing difficulty in navigating is nothing to be ashamed of. Secularism promotes an outward shell of steel, of confidence, of pride. We are given emotions by God to actually feel them; do not repress what God wants you to feel to heal. It's okay to acknowledge that our unknowns can be outright frightening. I often remind myself that God promised he will never abandon me. He has permitted evil to surround me, but God has not forsaken me. God has heard my pleas; he who is just knows what is best for me. I must believe God's Word and follow him.

He is my leader, he is my redeemer, he is my brother, and he loves me as I am, right now, unconditionally.

There comes a time for some in which they will eventually surrender to God's allowances, our plan. For some it's out of an obedience, for some the maintenance of sanity, and yet for others it may be a last-ditch effort to find relief from a relentless burden, by not giving in to the despair Satan desires for us, but having hope while submitting to God's will. Be still, find a quiet place, and know that he is God. We are his. In addition, our children and our grandchildren are his property. His children (who we call our own) have been loaned to us from God. We are to love them as God loves them, to teach them about our/their Father, Almighty God.

Do not waste another moment. Be gentle with yourself in your struggles and be gentle with your child who may be struggling while moving on to a new chapter. We are commanded to love God's children and teach them about God and show them how to share God's love with all his creation.

He was a natural athlete! He loved many different sports and his performance of each was loudly lived with coordinated movements, oftentimes engaging in great risks and always performing with infinite passion. It was pretty evident to all that he was most enamored with his trick riding abilities on his BMX push-bike! He carried both his exuberance and gorgeous grin mightily as he sailed down the city streets, maneuvering the winding roads without the slightest of fears. Anticipating the successful conquering of the unknown up ahead, he savored the ominous blind spots on the curves of his rides, which only gave him more satisfaction of the challenge. His left foot on the bike seat and his right foot on the handlebars, downward on that boulevard he would gracefully glide, just like a newborn eaglet leaving his nest.

This was a beautiful spring in Montana, and the neighborhood teenage girls would come to watch my son and his friends trick ride after school studying was completed. There were many afternoons, early evenings, and long weekends that the push bikes made their way around the city providing sheer pleasure and exercise for the boys and after-school entertainment for the girls. The girls were amazingly brave as they would lie on the ground in a row, and the boys would confidently sail in the air over the line of girls. I shake my head and smile.

Faith. Those girls conveyed unwavering faith in my only child and his loyal friends, just as I did. A spring of fun, one filled with laughter, boys meeting girls and girls sitting on the curb watching those hotshot boys perform with great assurance and passion, smirking from ear to ear. God had gifted me with a fun-loving, kind, handsome, intelligent young son that I was always very proud of. I smiled as I watched him enjoy his time with his friends and assured myself that I raised him well as I watched him treat others with respect. Yes, God gave me his son to raise, to love and teach; I am blessed.

As my son and I made our way to the middle school, taking our occasional two-mile jaunt after supper, we saw a friend on our way. She pulled over, and we visited a bit about the early evening, which many others were also out enjoying. This lovely friend was a teacher at the school I was working at; my position was to help young students with extra assistance. I was selected by the hiring board to facilitate, to be that bridge between the students and families and the school personnel. I was able to use my authentic desire to assist others who were in a needful place, to be a resource for some students and their families, giving them extra time to progress in their reading and in their math courses. It's my ingrained belief that all people created need a little extra care in some part of our being. God did not make us individually perfect. He commands us to share the gifts he gave to us individually with others who will be blessed. All gifts are commanded to be shared which equals one body, fully blessed.

This position of a liaison between the personnel and the families gave me a great selfless purpose and a continual satisfaction that I was able to share God's love with others through my actions and my words. It became my mission: sharing what I had been gifted with from God with others who were a little needful in a teensy area of their lives. I felt that I was being obedient to God, doing his work on his earth. I could shine God's light in sharing a smile with the students and families in addition to being responsible for fulfilling my assigned academic responsibilities at the school. I was so blessed. God answered my prayers in granting me the opportunity to be a servant, a needful place to live out my missionary services to others.

My calling! My own mission in the public-school system! Yes, my secret ministry! I am certainly feeling honored by God. He knows my heart and is much aware of my gifts to share and he has given me all that I have. It is to him I give the glory. My own area in the hallway was a welcome mat for the students to wave or stop over and chat. My couch became a gathering spot, my file cabinets quickly filling up with the files of the students rec-ognizing their advancements in reading and math in which they worked so tirelessly to perform. I was so happy to have these young students read to me; I always felt chosen and blessed. I smile as I see more students coming to my area to read to me and to show me how they have persevered to excel in their skills. I still smile, today, sixteen years later. I loved it when the students learned new words, expanding their vocabulary, reading with great accomplish-ment to me; today, others reading to me brings me great comfort.

My son and I exchanged our hellos, smiles and goodbyes, and some final smiles with our lovely new friend, and onward we traversed to the middle school and back to our home. My son acting hot-shot on his bike, me running behind him, smiling the whole way.

It was a gorgeous evening…no wind, which was a rarity, and this welcomed stillness soothed my soul. Seeing the beautiful sun setting in per-fection and noticing the life-filled buds on the trees and bushes as vibrant green, I didn't want this time to end. Why would we leave this beauty to go inside? To finish school assignments before Friday's graduation, that's why! My son decided it was time for him to return to his school assign-ments, and I decided to continue with enjoying the evening to resume walking and jogging, just like any other beautiful evening after supper; it was just too nice to go inside. I curled my fingers in a sweet goodbye and reminded him, "Two more miles and I'll be right back! We will go over all your final assignments and goals for the next three days when I get back."

"Will you also write down reminders of the things we need to do for sure before Friday's graduation?"

I had just turned forty and proclaimed quite loudly to my family and friends (even to the whole world I think!) that this surely was going to be the best year of my life. I was in tune with much, and I could feel it! Health and well-being were to be a top priority of many goals, recognizing I was way too sedentary over the cold winter months!

Maybe when all is revealed to me in heaven, it did turn out to be that, yes, it was the best year of my life. I no longer proclaim that which I think should be mine on earth. God's plan for our lives oftentimes is much different than what we see our life to be. We are not in control of most things in our lives—a fact that is hard for some to admit and embrace, actually by many, and quite frankly, by most. I was elated and truly quite thrilled about how several things in my life were looking at this point.

How dare that I be so bold to act like I should get what I want. Remembering those particular times I was behaving arrogantly in believing I had much figured out and believing I finally knew a lot of the answers I had searched long and hard for—acting as if I was my own god. Those beliefs of knowing and believing in some specific claims lasted a very short period of time. I should never exalt the abundances of my so-called successes and live as if it is my being and talents alone credited to find these treasures I thought I found. I must be humble. God is in charge of exultation. Reviewing those times, it's clear I wasn't giving God the glory for my…well, what I thought were my personal successes. This is a perfect example of "living in the world." I wasn't seeking God's favor; I was seeking my own favor through the world's eyes. I was living in the world with the world. My arrogance creeping upon me so stealthily—that's how Satan works in our lives, sometimes stealthily.

All that I have are gifts, blessings, and talents from God and I am commanded to share all that I possess. Sharing wasn't difficult for me; sharing with others all that I have always blessed me back. I treated my girlfriends to dinner to ensure that this "best year of my life" began with much love, joy, and fun. This evening would be memorable as it would be filled with many friends' love! I thought I felt love. I don't often stop to think of all the ways God blesses me, but when my friends congregated for my birthday dinner, I knew in their presence that I was blessed with love. I believe a lot of us in a lot of situations take much for granted and forget our Source.

Just two more miles. I would walk and jog intermittently as the blocks I would be on would be lengthening down to the grocery store, which was one mile down, and one mile back…and things always have to even out, right? Walk a block, jog a block, be able to jog as long as the blocks I walk on. Everything is measured, has to be exactly the same, black-and-white! Perfect finish to a beautiful spring day. Joy was in my heart, and peace was in my mind.

My only son, now settled at the kitchen table, just like any other evening after a jaunt after supper, was seriously focusing on his assignments for the coming days ahead. It's evident he had many feelings and thoughts this evening. Thinking about his fast-approaching graduation ceremony and events, he seemed a little distracted. Who wouldn't be? He was diligent, especially this evening, preparing for the last days at the middle school.

I placed eight quarters in my pocket and started down the road to the grocery store. Did I mention already that it's one mile down and one mile back? It would only take me a half hour to run down to the store. Getting in those two more miles would be healthy for me! Besides losing a few pounds, I was really feeling like I need to work on strength training! Everything seems to be congealing nicely in this little box I have in my brain about how things are working out and how well things will turn out in so many areas of my life.

The quarters jingle-jangled in my pocket. In that musical reminder, another joy-filled skip was added to my steps, grinning boldly as I ventured out to get a couple of sweet treats for my son!

Then finally after so much joy and fun, I would be calling today done. I would shower, smile, and crawl into my bed holding my pillow close and feeling certain that just like after every other night's sleep, I would awake refreshed and recharged. It always happens, and this would ensure that I would be at my best to be certain of the ability to assist the students at the elementary school and to continue to make "wonderful" the last couple school days with my son and finish up preparing for the graduation events and ceremony.

I had it all figured out.

That's an overly confident worldly statement, which is often used by many. It seems as if I have been using that same reassuring statement myself quite frequently.

So much has been accomplished and there's much to look forward to. Those good feelings, memories, and thoughts are even stronger as spring comes in with lots of sunshine, green grass, daffodils, and tulips carpeting all the lawns in our neighborhood. This life is simply beautiful. Everything is so amazing. Oh yes, and God is good.

His final year at the middle school was filled with many accomplishments and hard work: a time where friendships tightened, friends who were females discovered, growth in teamwork, encouragement to soar by loving intelligent educators, and growth in perseverance through trials. We were blessed to have people in our life that cared about our family and shared much love with us. We felt very blessed realizing the gift of having friends who shared the same values, morals, and ideals as our family did. I was a proud mother of a new teenager and was thankful to God that his formative years were filled with love and great selfless care from those who believed in God and set good examples morally, spiritually, mentally, emotionally, and physically. We are created to give God glory. In gratitude, I give God all the glory for these beautiful gifts we've been given. Thank you, our God.

It's important to deliberately take the time to be still, to listen to God. You will not hear God's wisdom and peace in the chaos of the world. Our culture has become a whirlwind of opposition, violence, technology, and busyness. It's necessary to take a moment and bring to your mind that all we have, our gifts, our blessings, our talents, the position we hold, the income we receive are all brought to us from God's grace. God is the giver of your gifts. It truly is imperative to recognize who is the God of your life. You will receive peace in the knowledge.

I didn't think that I took God's gifts to me for granted; I was attentive, and I was thankful. I am a sinner, and I know that in different times of my life, I have taken much for granted. I have taken God's blessings upon me for granted. My greatest gift from God is my son; I loved being around him. He was a person in my life with strength and an appealing disposition; he brought me great joy. We really had a pretty unique adventurous mother-son relationship; we still do, but today our relationship is very different from what it was, for many reasons. I am sure all relationships change. Whenever people are involved in anything that requires breathing, expect a change! There are always adjustments being made; honoring and being open to the changes bring health and well-being. Embrace and nurture your relationships. My son made me smile often, and it wasn't a secret that he was appreciative of my mothering skills, knacks, and my keen desire to be his loving mother. I knew I was one of the "fun" moms. I could tell by the friends my son cherished. I was his mother and, admittedly, not his friend. I was chosen to raise him and love him for our Father in heaven. I never expected to be his biggest fan when the boundaries were set and the curfews established. I wasn't in his world for him to like me. I was there to prepare him to soar—to soar with confidence, kindness, gratitude, and a multitude of other traits to grow and become the amazing man God expected. Most importantly, help him to get to know Jesus.

It's been approximately sixteen years since I took that "additional" two-mile jaunt to the store.

Sixteen years since I secretly placed those eight quarters into my pocket, jingling as I ran down the hill. I was on my way to get Reese's Peanut Butter Cups and a Snickers bar—treats for my son's final school days of eighth grade! He was never one to have a sweet tooth, but my thought was that he would think of the gesture as uncanny but know that I was congratulating him albeit in a very small way for all the accomplishments he has made. Besides, it's always fun for me, satisfying actually, to surprise others with the unexpected. I continue to live that way in surprising others with goodness and gifting generously with love.

Most often, that which is our core will shine through, no matter what. I felt so well, so at peace and joyful that beautiful evening of May 27, 2003. Sixteen years later, that cocky confidence, that continual laughter, that seemingly welcomed peace, that loud joy do not remain. Seemingly, I was knocked off my high horse, and God got my attention.

The year 2003 was the best year of my life; God was drawing me nearer to him.

I found myself in a strange place, sixteen years later; times so unfamiliar to me, grasping at straws and at every word the experts and know-it-alls proclaimed. Open to it all as I was wanting clarity and hastily seeking renewal, the results were a bombardment of information, and dark times of self-defeating exasperations. I was existing in this chaotic life of jumping into new, unfamiliar territories and navigating through the instructions of the so-called timeless motivational clichés of "new beginnings," "brand-new days," "positive words," "breathe in and breathe out," "new age must-reads," "eat this, don't think that," "keep your chin up," "be number one," "exercise this much," etc., which *promises human beings* wholeness. I made myself literally ill with the popular promises to wholeness and obtained no promised results of peace in any area I strove to make well. Let me confess to you that these ways of living I dove into, were definitely not the necessary antidotes for me to conquer the unsettling existence, nor were they the ultimately successful finds of the secrets to living in peace.

I attended Mass frequently all hours of the day, all days of the week. I took part in the offered sacraments (and continue to do so to this day) and simultaneously I was being tempted by Satan to seek a way of life that would prove to be "fun, filled with laughter, a loud peace perhaps," hence my seeking of more enthusiastic enjoyment outside of my Mass attendance.

I think Satan tries to disrupt our quiet times, which are times intended for us to hear the Holy Spirit.

I am speaking about resting in God's peace, God's joy, God's selflessness within me—living in God's image. Most often, yoga, essential oils on certain digits, ingesting a few or hundreds of supplements, journaling, acquiring eight hours of sleep, having a career that "you love," having a wide circle of friends, and so much more deceit simply do not make for a healthy peaceful existence for many, nor *me*. I tried living in a way that incorporated some of the above at times, all of the above at other times. I tried living in a way that was recommended by others and sworn by others to bring me peace, like jump in fast and hard and learn what it is that is bringing people you see all around in all areas of life, that peace and joy they are outwardly conveying. I really thought I wanted what others "had" or portrayed to have. Truthfully, I found what they had lived to convey is something that I did not want for myself. I was a broken hurting vessel, and not a thing in this earthly life could heal my brokenness, my days staggered with continual sadness. To you it may have been obvious I was grieving by what I divulged to you; however, I denied it. I closed every thought on any part of me attempting to open up to an acknowledgement of grief. Simply, many others' ways of grasping and maintaining a peace longed for definitely were not evidential successes for me. Just as each of us is uniquely created, I required a much different approach to wellness and peace. It was becoming very evident to me that we all are unique and we all require an individualized path to a particular peace, to comfort.

I come to share with you truths. An honest being to you, sharing my life. Feeling at God's peace, glorifying him for his timing and plans for me, accepting that his plans for me are the best. My hopes and dreams do not compare to what he has planned for me. I am excited to see what he has for me. New life has begun with his gifts granted to me through his servants, his children; they are doing God's will and have chosen to be obedient to God. I am aware, I am attentive; God continues to bless me. Thank you, Lord.

I have regurgitated those empty promises of "wholeness" through what was originally conveyed to me to bring health upon me. It was imperative that all falsities were removed so that truth and light would be allowed a place for growth within me, the temple of the Holy Spirit. The putrid soil, the stagnant refuse had to be removed to allow God's goodness to indwell. It's similar to sin; we must confess our transgressions, and we are given new life. This makes much sense to me. We try different things, ways of living that work for others, but we must remember that their path is not our path. Even others will bombard us with notions that fit their journey. Pause and remember that the journey God has you on is your own, not anyone else's. Be peace-filled even when you ache, and be assured you can embrace your very own one-of-a-kind journey. You are set apart. No one has, nor ever will, live your life. The reparation, a great light will be specifically provided to you from God. Those, my friends, are words of encouragement, light, and beauty. I have learned a great truth that holding inside of me others' transgressions toward me needed to be sounded, revealed out loud to escape a poison left upon me. I came to the crucial moment to upend the pretending that others' wrongdoings were to be accepted, resounded, and left—left behind. Share your hardships and pain with someone who has your best interests, someone who keeps confidences and encourages your continued growth toward pure peace. As individual as your fingerprints are is as individual your journey to peace will be…your own journey.

This book is most definitely not a self-help writing. It's an authorship wherein a part of it is naturally conveying that it's worth listening to the people God has placed in your life for your own and truly unique good (not for another's good). The timing and places are unexpected. There will come a period when you are prepared and genuinely ready to hear, then genuinely listen, to what someone has to share with you. It's about the importance of striving to reach a point to become open to another Christian's words about what it is that can be beneficial to your healing, a promotion of growth and love, ultimately receiving words, living them, and embracing the way to love as God loves. It's important to cherish your daily bread and do the work of Christ. There are obstacles for some to act on suggestions and words of others. Trust those who love Jesus Christ, trust those who God has placed on your journey; God wants you to have peace and solitude. You are his child. God is found in the quiet, not the loud busy chaos of madness. *Listen to him.* Have the courage to take necessary time to discern if who is in your life, who you spend time with, is genuinely who God is using in your life for your peace. Seek the wisdom of God our Father. This culture thrives in haste; you are set apart and responsible to be still and hear God's voice.

Trust in others who show you concern and seek to know if they truly have your best interests at heart. Surround yourself with believers. Know them by the way they conduct themselves, know them by their service and peace, know them by their fruit. Know them before you make yourself vulnerable. It's your position to be astute in choosing who you share your being with. At that realization of trust and goodness, be honest; share what is fully present on your walk. It is not worthwhile, nor will it prove to be a winning moment when you will deliberately keep something tucked and put away destructively in a dark place. We are assisted by others when that person God has chosen has the absolute truth. We cannot be helped in what's afflicting us when we are not truthful. God has beautifully provided and placed someone near to you who truly wants to help you evolve, to become that person God meant for you to be on this earth. Be open to his peace and love; these are God's ways. Travel and embrace your journey by keeping company with those who love God. It's paramount to goodness, peace, joy, and love—*true* goodness, *true* peace, *true* joy, and *true* love. *God is faithful. Seek him. Trust him. He cares for you.*

Care for yourself specially enough to seek an authentic peace. Care for yourself enough to learn what it is that you need to feel peace. Care for yourself enough to accept the love others have for you and accept the wisdom God gave to others to share specifically with you alone in helping you gain God's peace and kindness in your own life on this earth. God promised never to abandon us; he has an obedient servant who is close to you. Embrace his gift that he has provided for you to embrace as he prepares you to embrace that special being. Not only has God prepared a special place for you in eternity; he has prepared a special place for you to be present in receiving those he has sent to you. Be prepared for healing with genuine peaceful love. It's okay to be skeptical. You must be aware of who is in your life. Be still. He will show you his appointed servant. You will feel the moment in which to be open. You will feel his gentle touch even when you're sobbing in sorrow. A chosen servant made for you by our Creator has been chosen to be near to you as a gentle guide from God above. Open.

Blackness, eeriness—I am nauseated and trembling. I am hurting. I cannot move. I am immobile. Why am I aching? What is going on? My eyes are opening slowly, and it appears that I am on a hard surface. The sheets are quite cold and starkly white. Where am I? Am I in a hospital bed? Everything is quiet. There is no one around. Can I hear? I can't hear anything! Is something wrong? What is wrong? What is going on? Help! I am alone. I am in a terrified state of confusion. I look around this room, and I breathe in what smells like starch-pressed sheets. Everything looks and smells sanitary. I wonder in the silence as I lay all alone, "Am I in a hospital?" Why would I be in the hospital? No comprehension, blank, aware of nothing. I don't know what has happened, I don't know why I am immobile, I don't know why I hurt all over my body, but whatever has happened to me, please let me live long enough to raise my son. I know I have a son, but where is he? I knew that I had a child, that I did know. I don't know where he is. Did something happen to him? Where is he? Someone help me now! Help me! I don't know where I am. I don't know where I have been. I can't even comprehend the last moments I was cognizant of my surroundings. I am very confused. I am alone and this makes me sick. Where did I go tonight? I have no memory of the past hours and days. I will wait till someone comes to my room. They must have answers. Waiting, sort of panicking as I wait. I feel something lying on my chest on top of the sheets. I look down toward my feet. Everything appears sterile. I see what I believe is a newspaper lying on my chest. I can smell the print on the recently printed newspaper. Curiously, I lift up the newspaper and bring it close to my eyes. I cannot comprehend.

Astounded, shocked, sick to my stomach, disbelief…and every other sickening feeling you can imagine shakes me like I've never felt before. I am sick.

I would soon learn from a nurse making her rounds in the area where I was lying that this particular day that I became awake enough to notice something was amiss was the second day for me in the intensive care unit. The large newspaper article on the front page would expound on the immediate nausea I was feeling and initiate the unfolding of the mysterious plot as to why I was lying in a hospital bed.

FORTY-YEAR-OLD FEMALE JOGGER DELIBERATELY RUN DOWN BY SIXTEEN-YEAR-OLD BOY and

> *"Yes," he told the police officers who subsequently interviewed him, "I wanted to have sex with her corpse."*

Her. Is that "her" me? What is going on? I am quickly feeling faint and sick to my stomach, and a terrifying panic has begun to set in with a fury. I am terrified and feeling quite alone. That *her* is me, Ophelia Reim, and don't you remember that this year, her fortieth year of life, was going to be the best year of her life? Something dreadful has happened. I want to throw up.

I didn't immediately comprehend the facts; it took much time to evolve into a reality.

It was very strange. No one was with me when I awoke. No one sat by my bed to reach for my hand and gently explain where I was, why I was there, what was transpiring. I was left to be alone, again.

Didn't anyone recognize that I was beginning to come to a state of wondering where I was?

I am not fond of the person that placed that newspaper on my chest. I think that was cold, rude, and should have been avoided at all costs. It was an inappropriate action and an action I hope never happens to a victim again.

I would, at some point, not at all sure when, come to remind myself that sometimes the fallen angel Lucifer (more commonly known as Satan) is permitted by God's authority to act through others to cause evil, danger, and harm. God's Word proclaims that. I know that I have witnessed that and I have been subjected to evil throughout my life and I also am assured that God will never abandon me. He promised me that! I uttered these biblical truths to God, reiterating that I knew his Word and I would continue to believe his Word. I am his child, and this will not embitter me toward my Father, my Consoler, and my Lord Jesus Christ. He is bigger than this tragedy. With great faith and simultaneously experiencing severe panic, I chose to run to my Prince of peace. I prayed fervently to God. The more pain I felt, the more endurance I was granted to pray, and it took all I had to try to rest in him. The current unknowns I was absorbing led to a determination to continue to seek God. The more pain I felt, the more ardently I sought his face.

The loud noises of machinery and fluids continually flowing all over the room confirms my suppositions that I am in a hospital, somewhere. Where are the other people? Why don't I see anyone or hear anyone? Where are my mom and dad? Sometime later, I learned that I had suffered a traumatic brain injury and was subsequently reminded that not only did my parents not live nearby, but that in actuality, my mom and dad had passed away recently, my mom just two and a half months ago, and I had, in fact, attended her funeral out of state. Trauma of many sorts along with brain injuries are devastating in so many ways—ways that are known and so many unknowns to those who study the medical science and to the sufferers, the struggling survivors of the traumas.

When I have the means, the ability to share what I have, I am given so much unexplainable joy and peace in my soul from God. I feel blessed when I am able to share, to give. Sharing all that I have with my son and surprising him at times always brought me great joy and continual smiles. I knew well that my son was not a big fan of candy bars, but it was something small in gesture, and deep down, we both knew that it was more the effort and love I gave that he would appreciate and smile about, then it was about him indulging in the candy! It was the small but sincere gift that would bring him delight when I surprised him. We know each other pretty well; sometimes I think we know each other better than we know ourselves.

I will do what I can right now, live in this present moment, embrace today, and be the best that I can be right now; tomorrow has enough worries of its own.

I didn't see my girlfriend (whom I giggled with on that evening walk my son and I enjoyed together) at the elementary school on that supposed-to-be "tomorrow." I did see her at some point during my twenty-four days of the hospital stay split up in the intensive care unit, recovery and rehabilitation moves. She was one of hundreds who came to check in on me. I guess many people came to see me over that time period. I just have no memory of that.

Sometimes Satan is allowed to test us. God doesn't test us; the devil does that dirty plot. He is allowed by God to work evil. He uses others by tempting them. Sometimes they agree and sometimes they fight as hard as they can to deliver themselves from the ugly ploys of Satan. I have always had a great affinity toward growing nearer and nearer to God. Always. That doesn't mean I didn't falter and fall flat on my face and beg for forgiveness and mercy! I choose the Lord as my light and my salvation. The Lord is my God.

I reiterated once again to the evil one, "No, this incident orchestrated by you does not diminish my faith in my Creator and my deep love for him." Those words are constantly on my tongue.

God was with me, and he promised me that he would never abandon me. This is spoken in his Word. "Lord, I continue to believe in you." By now you probably have gathered that I never did return home that beautiful evening to surprise my soon-to-be-graduate with the Reese's Peanut Butter Cups and the Snickers bar. Sadly, I never even made it to the grocery store.

"Have no anxiety," his Word instructs us of that command. No matter our circumstances, no matter if there's bleakness or the demise of a plan, we are to have no anxiety and expect to be fed and clothed just as the birds of the air live in freedom knowing God will always take care of them. God has equipped us. He cares for us. Have faith in his Word. Oh boy. I can read that, I can say that out loud, I can share that wisdom with the suffering, shout it out to others loudly so they grasp that truth, but today, I am feeling lost, scared, and alone. I am in need of some revival, of great blessings and peace to my soul. I am requiring something good.

If you're at all human, you will have said or will say, "I will do this," "I will do that," "I will see you then," "I will see you there next week, next month, next year," "We will do this and that and claim this and claim that," etc. No! We are commanded to live presently and know that our tomorrows are not a promise to us in his Word. Death is promised; life is not. Live accordingly. We live in this world believing it's important to have things to look forward to, to have that which we feel will benefit us in some way. God's plan has the final word. Be content with your todays and do your best to be the person today who God has made you to be.

I learned over time that the sixteen-year-old boy operating the Dodge Ram who intentionally hit me from behind didn't only want to simply kill me; he wanted to sexually assault my corpse.

His passenger told the police that he personally did not believe that the driver, his friend of *eight* long years, a current classmate, would actually do what he said he wanted to do. After the near-fatal strike and the dragging of my body for twenty-five feet underneath the operator's truck, the passenger pleaded with the driver to take him home.

The passenger maintains in his words to the police that he didn't believe the driver would jump a curb with the Dodge Ram and ultimately go up on to a city street sidewalk and hit me at thirty miles per hour. Trust me, when I could, I always found a sidewalk to walk and jog on. I was uncomfortable running on a road. I have seen others do it all the time. I shudder. As you are aware, it can be very dangerous and, quite clearly, almost deadly walking on a sidewalk most anywhere, even in the center of Montana, typically referred to "rural," which has been coined in various regard as "the last best place."

This was my quiet place, my arena in which to get things accomplished, a place I considered "my" sacred place, to just "be," in the peace of the early evenings, walking, jogging, and praying. My parents had recently passed away, and on these evening jaunts, I was able to pray, seeking to find great peace; it came to be a place I would always find deep solace. It was a comfort to me after eating supper and right before bedtime; this was my routine. This was my precious time to feel comfort and joy, to pray, a time for reflection, a time for thanksgiving and lifting up numerous supplications to our God. This was sacred time in a sacred place, my serenity.

Prior to being struck, Dick, the operator, and Pat, his passenger, had been driving around, enjoying a springtime evening in the area where I was praying and enjoying spring weather myself. They reported to the police that they had aborted the attempted deliberate homicide on two occasions, only moments before the near-fatal hit. United in the successful strike, they immediately confirmed to the police the desires Dick had shared with Pat, of his hopes of sexually assaulting my corpse.

That successful strike was at the location of their high school's tennis courts; the high school was located immediately across the street, where they were completing their sophomore year of high school.

Two previous attempts were halted as they saw vehicles driving in the vicinities of where I was jogging; obviously, not wanting to be seen, they hid, tucked away in different areas of their high school, waiting for their next opportunity wherein they would be able to claim that this strike was "the completed mission, the successful strike."

Within a few hours, Pat was cleared of any charges. By clearly convincing the authorities conducting the investigation and all charging entities, that he "truly didn't believe that Dick would follow through with the attempted deliberate homicide and subsequent rape," *no charges would be filed against Pat.* I am certain you know how I feel about that decision made regarding the passenger. The passenger who was picked up sometime earlier in the evening contributed gas money for the joyride and rode shotgun with Dick throughout the entire unfolding of the plans Dick shared with Pat to run me over, killing me, throwing me in the back of the truck, and sexually assaulting me.

Would you continue riding in that truck if someone shared with you the hopes of his evil ways, dodging other vehicles to remain anonymous, ducking into a parking lot? I hope not.

I had reasonable thoughts, spurning skepticism, and a higher education of affirming my beliefs and thoughts and great wisdom about the quick decisions made by those responsible to charge Pat with a crime. I will have the never-ending disagreement with these decisions made by investigative officers and a county attorney's office. My opinion forever stands: Pat is guilty of being an accomplice to an attempted deliberate homicide. Those words sting. They are strong words, and participating in that joyride that evening was a decision made completely by Pat alone, a decision to continue on in the passenger's seat throughout the completion of the desires Dick shared with Pat.

I am not in agreement with the short and vague reports composed by the police officers and investigators which were filed with the county attorney's office, the entity which would be in authority to charge this passenger with a crime. I am not in agreement with anyone who worked the case, the judge who judged the crime, etc., including that the passenger was in no way chargeable. Just like many other cases of confusion and skepticism, no satisfaction or closure, a victim does not have a right to question, visit with, share her thoughts and feelings with, or state her opinion regarding the fact that a passenger verbalizing to officers that he agreed to go along for a "joyride" with his friend of eight years was immediately cleared of any wrongdoing. The passenger admits to police his contribution to the gas fund for the evening joyride and participated fully in the driver's whims.

This passenger made a conscious decision over possibly forty minutes, a holding-on effort to joyride in his friend's truck, holding tight in his seat through two of their aborted attempts to strike and kill me, making a conscious decision to continue on and to actively participate in the joyride in that Dodge Ram driven by his close friend of eight years, maintaining his front seat position during the *third* ominous strike, which was intended to end my life but only severely disabled me.

Pat made many decisions in that short period of time while the plot Dick had conjured up was beginning to unfold. Pat's decision to "stand by" his friend in the completion of this plot (well, literally seated inches away next to him in the truck riding shotgun) was clearly evident and real. Pat fully participated in a gruesome and evil event in which he knew was meant to end my life. Dick told him so. Well, that's what the passenger reports to the police. Well, that's what the reports say.

As you can feel and hear, I am not pleased with many outcomes in this attempted deliberate homicide. I often wonder how other people would feel in my place. It doesn't matter. I remind myself my feelings and thoughts are valid and it's my right to have my opinions.

The passenger's lack of an apology for the abominable association he freely chose to be a part of conveys, loudly to me, cowardice and a huge lack of remorse. After being an actively involved, excited spectator to the attempted deliberate homicide in undeserved freedom, the passenger fled the city to begin a new existence. How does one flee with such darkness following? Why is it that some can't see their wrongs, admit their guilt, apologize, and repent? Lack of charity maybe? Lack of morality? Clearly, they aren't sorrowful; otherwise apologies would be made. The lack of an apology astounds me and leaves me breathless. I must wonder, who raised this boy? One can't move on in a healthy livelihood by ignoring past transgressions. One must apologize and repent; that's what God's Word commands. Just like one can't move on in a productive livelihood by trying to forget, ignore, and escape, the new realities of life changes after being the victim of an attempted deliberate homicide. I have tried to flee the truth and horrors of my victimization, a detestable crime that has for a very long time paralyzed me in many ways. I truly live sickened by the actual crime, the plot of preparing to make this successful for the occupants, the families who have shown no sorrow and felt their boys were victimized, brushing by me in the courthouse, holding tightly on to her rosary. People always will and always have tried to run away, ignore, put in the past, and repress the crimes they were involved in. The darkness remains; it's just below where they attempted to hide it, where they think they are tucking it away. Darkness isn't ever tucked away. Its effects will randomly appear at an unexpected time, needing to be dealt with once and for all. Darkness is only lifted when it's brought into the light.

The investigative reports by many officers give no indication that the passenger made an attempt to warn me (please recall, this passenger admitted to the police that this final near-fatal attempt to kill me was *the vehicle's two occupants' third attempt to run me down*). The passenger would in no way make even a miniscule attempt to help me in some way, to help me become aware of my impending doom. This passenger did not yell out to me; he simply refrained from screaming out the window. He did not attempt to try to honk the horn of the truck, nor did he make any attempt to redirect nor complicate the driver's plan to kill me. Pat made no effort to interrupt a crime he knew full well was soon to be committed. As sure as he participated in hiding out in various areas around the high school, a crime was going to be committed.

To me, and I would surmise to most people in the world, it is highly probable that the outcome and severity of the strike would have been drastically minimized or the successful third strike completely diminished if the passenger would have had the morality to consider my welfare. No one can refute that his many inactions show very loudly that he had no regard for my life whatsoever.

At the very least, this passenger had a moral obligation to scream to me of the impending harm he was made privy to. Window up, windows down, it doesn't matter. There is no report of him screaming out loud. Most human beings who have even somewhat of a conscience would have warned me during the first attempt of the near-fatal hit. It's very clear, the passenger decided to continue to remain in the Dodge Ram until the near-fatal hit. That's extremely disturbing to me, and I believe that this passenger should have been charged as an accomplice to this horrific crime. He, in no way, should have been deemed innocent by anyone whatsoever. I find him guilty.

I will expound later in this book on the relationships that were maintained at this time, relationships which I feel strongly had an impact on the determination of involved authorities not to charge this passenger. With very little delving, I have discovered that the web that encapsulates all those involved is thick. It may not appear as such, as a noninvolved reader to the articles published in the newspaper, but I dug a little, and it gets pretty disturbing. You, too, will recognize a common practice of secrecy, sweeping much under a rug, statuses, those kinds of things, where the truth just was never important enough to be shared by anyone involved.

I am an educated woman. I graduated from an amazing university excelling in the studies of criminal justice and psychology; however, I chose not to proceed in the field of law enforcement. I have worked in many facets of law enforcement and hold much respect for honest police work. I come from law enforcement lineage and I proudly back the blue. I have the evidence in reports regarding this passenger, and I fiercely condemn the passenger for his association to this crime. He would be serving time if I would have been involved in the responding and the investigation of this ugly

attempted deliberate homicide. This is victim bru-
tality. There were many components (people and
relationships) to this wrongly made decision to
vindicate this passenger. I stand up for myself, the
justice system errored. This may be an appropriate
time to iterate something. I feel it's a good time
to make a point. It's important that if you are a
major decision-maker in any regard that involves
an acquaintance, a friend, a relative, a friend of a
friend, an acquaintance of a relative or a friend—
you get my point, always uphold your oaths.

If there is even the slightest of possibilities
that someone who will be making a decision of
any sort involving a criminal justice matter/civil
lawsuit, who may be even in the most miniscule of
levels of acquaintanceships or of a low-level party
to an association, it should be mandatory for that
person to recuse themselves of any involvement on
any level of decision-making. It's imperative if one
is unable to be impartial in any degree because of a
relationship or an association of *any sort* to make a
moral decision to take leave of making a decision,
to recuse yourself from your position. It is commanded for you to be honest and impartial if you
are to follow through on making any decision.

Caustically, I was ordered to pay the passenger's
legal fees in a civil lawsuit wherein he was named
a defendant. The passenger was quickly dismissed
by a well-known local district court judge—a judge
whose family had decades of roots in the area with

many associations, in many different circles. I am going to talk about that just a bit later in the book. Unable, for so many years, to keep trying to outrun the undeniable truths that the driver's actions and the excitable cheerleading passenger have placed upon me physically, mentally, emotionally, socially, and spiritually, after sixteen years of running from this tragedy, I surrender. I accept the occupants of the striking vehicle's evil ways and desires to kill me. I have begun to embrace all that has become new and foreign from before the strike, the pains, the immobility, the confusion, the PTSD, the anxiety, the depression, the many traumatic brain injury repercussions, and all the many symptoms and ramifications that are party to the many diagnoses. I have come to a point wherein pretending I was not affected, always trying to hide the damages that occurred, was in no way a healthy existence, pretending "well-being" created much hardship. I was lying, therefore, sinning. All that I was doing was only prolonging the beginning to a recovery that deep inside I so needed and wanted. I ran from the truth, just as the passenger ran from the truth. I was living a lie, living pretentiously. I accept the demise and walk toward the healing.

It was a warm spring early evening. The sun was warm and bright, a very pleasant time I recall. I am quite certain those boys joyriding in that Dodge Ram had their windows rolled down as they scouted out where they would run me over, hoping that no one else was around to witness their evildoings. That's exactly what they were hoping to do (find a certain block, alley, or roadway without a witness to their morally revolting unwrapping of their ugly plan). As the night got darker, the first two strike attempts were successfully aborted in the area of the high school they both attended. The third and final attempt at the successful strike was deemed a success; however, there were people that came to my aid. These people just weren't in the vehicles these criminals were successful in avoiding.

(I want you to know that I in no way have the ability to make this information up. This information is retrieved from the police reports I am privy to, the local and national newspapers, and public information which the internet screams out loudly the information regarding this crime.)

The two-toned brown Dodge Ram hit me from behind at the speed of thirty miles per hour, deliberately driven up over the curb and onto the sidewalk where I was speed walking. The truck's bumper and metal attachments pummeled into my body, beginning at hip level going downward into my left thigh. My back, neck, and head careened rapidly backward onto the Ram's hood. As the speed of the truck continued on at thirty miles per hour, I was thrust forward onto the cement and gravel alleyway, four feet from the hood with my forehead sustaining the forced blunt connection with the ground, the tragic impact clearly written upon my forehead for all time. A raised hematoma, a shade of blue. As the metal attachments protruded into my left hip, my body was held tightly to the underside of the truck, being dragged approximately twenty-five feet across the asphalt and gravel near their high school's tennis courts. Eventually detaching from the Dodge Ram, my lifeless body was left alone for dead. It must have been a very dark, horrific ride. I am thankful to God that I was unconscious during that ride underneath that truck. At this point, I have just about all the tragedy I can handle. That unauthorized near-death ride left me broken and desolate in every way one can begin to imagine. The Word of God reminds us that there are seasons in life. It's evident my existence that beautiful evening was hated by these two young boys for reasons unbeknownst to me; this was most definitely not a season for "life and peace" in their lives on May 27, 2003, at about 8:46 p.m., just before dusk.

Those two sophomore boys, they left me there alone. Pat, the passenger, he wanted to go home to his mother, and Dick, the driver, was planning to return to the tennis courts to throw my body into the back of his truck and rape me after taking Pat to his house. According to the many police reports, this was that big moment when Pat decided that he had dipped his toes in a bit too far for his comfort level. Apparently, Pat, who obviously willingly participated in the unfolding of Dick's New Year's Resolution number 1 to its horrific, devastating almost-deathly finish, has seen and heard enough. It's obviously a little late—Pat's agreed to accompaniment and the unrefuted presence of being an accomplice to Dick were securely established. Pat pleaded with Dick to take him home, begging and pleading. Before Pat left the now-damaged Dodge Ram, he explained to Dick that he would not divulge to anyone what they were just involved in. My thought was "Who raised these two boys to behave as such?" This behavior is not acceptable.

The nearby homeowners had seen me jog by their home. They were familiar with me as running by their home was a regular occurrence. Both were terrified and yelling to each other from different windows in the house as they witnessed the Dodge Ram lined up point-blank with my body on the sidewalk. Godly people in word and deed, they ran outside to determine exactly what was transpiring. They recognized it was my life that was expiring as they covered me gently with Grace's home-made quilt and waited with me for the ambulance to arrive. They didn't leave my body. They had a rich goodness within; they had morals. God gifted them with beautiful qualities, and they shared their gifts with me. The students practicing a sport at the high school across the street came to my aid and held my hand until the first responders arrived. God sent his angels to surround me. I speak kindly of these angels because I read in the police reports what these bystanders did for me. Recognizing the goodness in others is paramount to well-being. The students from Dick's and Pat's high school didn't see the attack, but they were astute and selfless and immediately responded to hearing my agony and cries for help. There truly are people who live by God's word. They came to comfort me (so the reports say); they, too, did not leave my body. I thank their parents for raising these children with morals, with charity and service.

Law enforcement called my son and his father, eight blocks up the road: "There has been a terrible accident." At that point in time, it was a hit-and-run and, shortly thereafter, an attempted deliberate homicide.

My son and his father were now at the hospital seeing my lifeless body on the stretcher being pushed around inside the emergency room. They were quickly approached by the on-duty chaplain, who would look into my son's eyes and inform him that "your mother may not make it." I read these words, and my heart aches. You know what happens when your heart aches, don't you? A part of your being is dying. Pay attention to that gross pain, that intensifying ache. That ache is the palpable remnant of a sting. We are stung thousands of times in our lifetime and there is only so much sting a heart can afford before it stops beating. Please choose carefully who you spend your time with, who you allow into your heart. Be protective of your heart. Your time is precious and your heart more sensitive than you know. Allow me to elaborate. We will return to the gruesomeness and immorality of the crime wherein I was the target in just a few minutes.

When you ignore me, I feel that sting. Personally, I have a very big heart, I am sensitive, and I have compassion for all creation that is immeasurable. I ache when animals are killed on the road, whether someone killed them purposefully or if they were in the wrong place at the wrong time and the driver could not safely avoid the animal to save its life.

When I am stung, I am aching considerably, and as the sensation of the sting is so real to me, as I write this to you to share a little about me personally, I ache and I cry because that sting goes very deep within me.

So as I share the aches of the stings in my life, a part of me is literally dying.

When you slight others, marginalize another, when you brush by a person in your disrespect or avoid a disabled person (for whatever your excuse may be), you create a sensational sting. Our hearts will only survive so much of the stinging. There will come a time when your contribution of slights toward others will in effect kill them. When you are not interested in learning about and exploring how disabilities affect your loved one, you choose to show no interest in that life, and that stings your beloved. When you are not interested in realizing the immense difficulties the medical experts have to successfully treat the hundreds of symptoms a PTSD patient (your friend, your brother, your parent) endures, your stings are felt. Your lack of interest, your lack of concern, your lack of association create an unforgettable sting—stings that will lead to the receiver isolating. In essence, your ignorance of a loved one's troubling issues that are debilitating often appears as an apathy which compels the sufferer to isolate further. This is a sidenote. There is so much more for me to share on this particular topic, but not in this book.

The list of stings is infinite. As you ponder this insert, you will become aware that stings come in many forms and are delivered in many ways. I inserted this spontaneously urging you to be informed. Throughout this book, the Holy Spirit is gently nudging me. Readers, I want you to know how, when you avoid, ignore, slight, or do anything that isn't of God, it hurts others so very deeply. This sidenote will remind you to be aware, to make known to you that you are responsible for creating a sting. A human being is only able to live through so many of these stings. I identify a sting as a loud injustice causing intense pain, an indignity intentionally produced by none other than God's creation—a creation he named "good." We must all be cognizant of how we are treating one another. We have all fallen short, and it's never too late to repent and treat God's creation with care. There's no pain at death. Those stings omitted the beat of your heart. You were experiencing death at the times you felt those stings. Stop the stings, do what is right and good, and when you offer to help others in whatever situation they may be needing some assistance, don't abandon them because it's "too hard." Don't leave those others behind.

This would be a "wait and see" situation. The physicians who were specialized in the several specific areas of necessary care were on-call and would be arriving shortly at the hospital. Triaging, the emergency room personnel did what they could do for me to maintain as much stabilization as possible. The hospital corridors were bustling this Tuesday evening, but many sets of eyes were monitoring me as I lay on a gurney in and out of consciousness. The conscious moments were filled with excruciating back pain. Of course, there would be pain. I survived four pelvic fractures among many other injuries; of course my back was in severe pain—the severest, darkest pain I had ever been introduced to. There was no relief. I could not be moved in any fashion until attending physicians made assessments. Soon the three specialized providers would arrive, calculate the extent of injuries, and determine which physician would need to address firstly the severest medical issue. I knew God cared for me. I knew that he asked me to trust him by casting all my anxieties and darkness on him, but really, in the short moments of consciousness, I had no idea what was transpiring, and at that moment God wasn't on my lips; there was nothing on my lips, my heart, or my mind. All was dark. There would be a priority of care, assessments, and interventions.

In this darkness, nothing existed. Sheer emptiness. I couldn't hear, I couldn't see, and I was immobile. I don't think that death is that way, but what I do know, death is a mystery. Presently unconscious and intermittently conscious, the only words I can recall hearing in those two lost days was someone saying that I would no longer be intubated. Nauseated and very much unalive, I fell into unconsciousness.

It was imperative that the bleeding be stopped in my perineal area; a metal attachment on Dick's truck sliced deeply into my body and the blood transfusion became necessary. I had worried about receiving another's blood throughout my life. I was concerned of disease and drugs in others' blood. Sometimes we have no control over things in our lives…a great deal of our lives we are not in control of. I learned some lessons very quickly—big lessons.

There would be a delay in the preparation for the necessary vascular surgery as this surgeon would need a clearance from the osteopathic surgeon who would first make an important decision on the determination that my spinal cord would not be in any way jeopardized by any bodily manipulations to be made by the vascular surgeon to repair my perineal area in addition to any other potential dangers to me. Clearance was finally granted hours after my arrival to the emergency room, and the vascular surgeon would begin to repair my perineal and also give immediate attention to the large gaping hole in my left side below my rib cage that, too, was contributing to the continual loss of blood—another area where attachments on Dick's truck deeply sliced into my flesh. I can't imagine what went on underneath of Dick's truck for those twenty-five feet. I am quite certain that's a blessing that I do not know. I now wonder if Dick and Pat could hear my body being thumped around underneath Dick's truck during their joyride. Did I scream? Did they hear me scream? That information was not denoted in the police report I guess. What does it really matter? At different times when I am thinking about the crime, new questions arise that I have. It's all part of healing, I remind myself. Some things I don't need to know; after all, some information is not helpful to my healing. Some information is just that…just information. I remind myself that I go forward always and also remind myself it's okay to ask questions even if I have no one to answer them. Blessed, I thank God that parts of my brain are still working. I don't take brain function for granted. My brain is so precious to me. It sustained great injury, but I am gentle with what remains. I haven't always been gentle with what remains, but I am today, that's what matters. A victim can at times be hard on herself and have expectations that are impossible to attain. Becoming gentle with this manipulated being has taken much time, but the time is now to accept and embrace this changed Ophelia.

This one-and-a-half-inch fleshy hole in my side was doused with water and a disinfectant and given the attention of a tightly fit drain tube to relieve the area of probable infection and to remove as many of the fluids possible from accumulating at the injury site. With flesh now closed, a multitude of scans, imaging, and examinations were ongoing to determine in what order it was necessary for the triage team to work their proficiencies, adding more experience to their years of expertise. The loss of my innocent life was what these providers were attempting to prevent.

Some of the people God created make a choice to attempt a deliberate homicide, a self-proclaimed "valiant" attempt to stop a beating heart. Others created by the same God embark on a moral feat to do all they can to try to reverse that attempt and promote continued life.

In essence, some will try with all that is within them to get your blood to stop circulating. Others carefully add a stranger's life blood to the victim's remaining blood that had been left circulating to try with all their being to navigate through all that's required to try to help a victim maintain the status of "life."

All individuals involved were created by God, but in God's gift of free will to his children, each made a deliberate choice and decided to use what they have, for evil or for good.

These individuals are all a part of God's creation. His very own children, his two young boys, have chosen immorality by attempting to end an innocent life. Many seek morality in attempting to sustain a life.

One has chosen the darkness, one has chosen the light. One has chosen selfishness, one has chosen selflessness. One has chosen masterfulness, one has chosen humility.

Satan tries so hard to create a worldwide darkness and death all around us. Sometimes we fall, sometimes we find great strength to ascend that evil desire. I, too, have been tempted, fallen, and guilty. Thank you, God, for giving me the opportunity to repent of my sins. Thank you, God, for your mercy, your grace, and your unending love for me, your child.

Rewind: The best year of my life,
I proclaimed to the world.

Play: I lived believing I was innately (and
expected that for all time) vibrant and energetic.
I was filled with life, exuberant laughter, I was
on fire for our Lord and on fire for the life he
afforded me! Healthy, extroverted, living largely
with enthusiasm and forever smiles, genuine
guffaws, I was feeling on top of the world.

Pause: Victim of an attempted deliberate homicide.

Forward: Diagnoses of a traumatic brain injury (with its many unpredictable and surprising repercussions), PTSD (with its many and oftentimes debilitating symptoms and effects), anxiety and depression, chronic nerve and joint pain, disc degeneration, chronic neck pain and decreased mobility, arthritis, inflammation.

Stop: Immobility, confusion, endless pain, constant hardships, and continual losses.

Fast-forward: "Surely God is my salvation; I will trust and not be afraid. The Lord, the Lord himself, is my strength and my defense; has become my salvation" (Isaiah 12:2).

Play: Viewed as an overcomer in many ways, an encourager to self. Reminder to do all I can to stay as grounded as I am possible on this journey and know for certainty that I continue to maintain God's gifts and talents that he wants me to share. Do everything in my power to find a serene and level balance, just as God has prepared for me to hold. Persevering in all that is good, believing in an enormous victory, which is God's peace.

Final stop: Surrender. Accept God's blessings. Rejoice.

Unbelievably, the road rash is difficult to look at, but the pain and continual discomfort is again becoming unbearable. I feel an assortment of distinct pains, unrecognizable aches and stings. I never knew that my body had so many parts that could be afflicted with pain. The traumatic brain injury obviously isn't visible to my eyes, but that large lump on my forehead signifies to me something tragic. Daily, this large lump, the flesh encircling this nodule, slightly discolored, is a reminder to me that someone wanted me to be deceased and worked very hard to try to accomplish his number one resolution on his New Year's Resolution Comp assignment with his friend of eight years in tow. Not surprising to you, I'm sure, many hours of a day, a daily occurrence, my existence is filled with tearful sadness and anger. I will not lie. This victimization tears me apart. Hanging my hat on the many responsibilities I juggled in my life in all areas, always being the stickler for organization, holding long-standing bragging rights of an impeccable memory, astute in prioritizing and organizing, closest attention to detail you won't outwin, truth be told, I surrender to the inability to do what I was able to do before the incident. Albeit obstinate and reluctant, I learned and accepted that the TBI of my frontal lobe permanently obstructed highly executive cognitive skill functioning. No matter how much therapy, practice, health, prayer, those skills I once bragged of *will never return...*

Those brain cells are dead. The inability to complete the simplest of tasks to place documents in date order has left me in tears and in confusion. Lest I will confidently display and embrace acceptance, adjustment, and a realignment.

All have many moments of trying to recall something. Most often, what is trying to be recalled is recalled. "Oh yeah," we would say in recalling that information. It gives us satisfaction. Our brain is a wonderful operation. Feel blessed, be grateful to God for his wonderous intricately woven being he created in you. TBIs often leave a sufferer with the sad news that oftentimes, the recollection will never come. That "Oh yeah" isn't realized very often. Short-term memory loss is a hard difficulty to endure.

I had always taken great pride in being able to call people by name without hints or stammering, remember sixteen digits of a card, remembering many people's phone numbers, birthdays, addresses, the random information that was stored and retrieved very easily. I never took that ability for granted; it's just strange how it all changed in a couple of minutes.

Vanished!

Those wonderful God-given abilities and talents are not available to me any longer. God had other plans for me, allowing Satan to tempt me, harm me, attempting to take away my strong and loyal devotion and adoration to Jesus Christ.

God knew what was, and is, in store for me. I am in agreement with God's goodness. God makes beautiful what he allowed Satan to try to make not so beautiful. God prevails. Some days I really do believe God makes good out of Satan's attempts to destroy.

The human within me has a difficult time adjusting to the bouts of lack of concentration, little to no sequencing ability, toils of being easily distracted, surviving short-term memory loss. I have often found myself going around in circles trying to complete a task. It caused a great deal of pain and sometimes hardships, but today I shake my head and carry on. It's an ongoing ordeal to accept the loss of such important abilities that made my life easy in so many areas. I once found these talents to be innate. I may find myself stopping where I am at, literally standing in one place, and do all that I can to concentrate without any noise in the background. Still to no avail I am unable to do what I am attempting to complete. It's important to be gentle with oneself when adaptations must be implemented to follow through on responsibilities, loving myself enough to do what is necessary to live peacefully in this fallen world. It may take me much longer to complete a task at this time in my life, or forget a few times what my end goal is, but eventually on some occasions, I actually do figure it out and complete what I have begun. If I am unable to complete a task, I forgive myself and do my best to be gentle with myself. I try not to chastise myself, a vessel that is hugely compromised.

Acceptance: higher order/executive functioning = new procedures required. It's highly probable that on many tasks, there will be incompletions. Asking for others to help me has become commonplace, and I am not as ashamed and embarrassed as I was several years ago. I am receiving many lessons in humility.

While hospitalized, not certain what day it was in relation to the incident, I had an appointment with the speech therapist who was assigned to my case to determine the extent of the compromises stemming from my traumatic brain injury. She addressed me, iterating that apparently, some people were noticing that I was repeating myself. I ended the appointment abruptly in anger and in fear. There is no way there can be something wrong with me. I cry as I write today, fighting so hard with others, trying to convince them that I in no way suffered a TBI. In her evaluation of me, she attempted to convey with courage that in fact, yes, my brain had been adversely affected by the attack and that, yes, one very evident key to that determination was that I keep repeating myself. Scared and sad, I told her that she was wrong and that she was never to come back to my hospital room. She never returned.

I don't know if I had a replacement for this therapist that was trying to complete her work or if personnel decided that it wasn't necessary to further evaluate. TBI sufferers experiencing PTSD are set apart; agitation and anger are at the forefront. I kept reassuring myself and everyone around me that I did not have any damage to my brain, there was no brain injury, only a lump on my forehead that would dissolve. I reminded those who came to visit me that my brain's ability to think, solve, organize, and remember is impeccable! In all my assertions, my loudness, and my fright, I learned that I was wrong, the speech therapist was incredibly right. I was wrong again. The lump on my forehead remains. There are many things that happened during my hospital stay that I am not in agreement with. Looking back, I was bombarded with appointments with providers and therapists constantly in and out of my hospital rooms. Constant activities, constant traffic, everything was whirling. Noise, noise, and more noise.

I have to share something with you that is not easy to say. The times were dark. I was living in a constant terrifying state. I felt under attack at all times. It was imperative for me to leave the city and all the reminders that constantly bombarded me and stole my peace every waking moment. Everything in that city and in various parts of that state reminded me of this horrific crime these two young boys created and also brought to my mind constantly all the people I believe were… Never mind, I will share that later. For right now, I want you to know that my healing has progressed most notably since I have left that city in Montana. I was in peril for many years. I required a quiet place for healing to begin. Finally, I am beginning to heal. I will tell you that one cannot heal surrounded by remnants of evil, and I am not speaking solely about those directly involved in the attempted deliberate homicide. God has saved me. God nudged me for a long time to physically leave that area behind. I did, and now the healing has begun. I thank God for much.

For many years I had denied any damage to my brain. I had been on the run from my body's truths and my brain's truths. I had pretended for years that I was safe, I was healthy, and well, that whatever some people had said about the obvious cognitive changes and what actually had resulted from that vicious act, it certainly didn't affect me! I vehemently denied I had PTSD, a traumatic brain injury, anxiety and depression, and (attempting to hide) the hundreds of symptoms that accompany the many ugly, stigmatizing, and outright marginalizing diagnoses. The physical ailments were more difficult to hide, and today there's no denying that my body suffers. I lied, I fibbed, I had always pretended that nothing had changed after the tragedy. The physical disabling pains were, and are, undeniable; I can no longer do anything to hide those pains. These physical implications were the beginning of me no longer having the ability to hide my truth of pain. The results of many fractures certainly have a lasting impact on me. Stretch, reposition, sit, stand, kneel, lie down, walk, reach, and continue that repetitive cycle hundreds of times a day to at least try to reduce that unrelenting pain. Move. Perpetual motion. I wear myself out daily trying to remove my pains. Every miniscule moment I live, I am acutely aware of. It was apparent I was not a survivor of an attempted deliberate homicide that received a miraculous healing. I am not the survivor who now runs marathons, and my life suddenly turned glorious. These events may happen truly for others—not many but possibly for some. The array of severe injuries in so many areas of physical, social, mental, emotional, and spiritual functioning that I have truly sustained does not allow me opportunities to pull myself up and conquer the world! My life has changed dramatically, but what is most important is that God has heard my cry in my supplication. He is blessing me with his peace. I don't offer up my supplications for the wealth the world searches for. My prayers are concise: "Please take me to heaven when I die. While I am on earth, please give me your peace. Amen."

For sixteen years I continually made a proclamation to myself: "I am not a victim and I am not going to be a victim. I will not take medications for pain or for the symptoms of the many other diagnoses or issues related to the deliberate attempted homicide. I am invincible and I will live that out."

I am strong and can begin to heal with my own ideas. I will handle this my way. I had a mission to portray an invincibility to a near-death criminal act. I wanted to show the world that others' betrayal of me will not affect me in any regard. Besides, I want to be an individual who others will want to emulate to find healing.

I was a stranger to all the ramifications of being victimized by this type of event, but I wasn't going to admit that this tragedy had beaten me up and changed my life. I guess, yes, you could say that I was prideful, I was stubborn, I know how others are looked at many times in the treatment sought for various repercussions of illnesses, pains, and brokenness. I am stronger than the evil that was plotted. I don't want people to judge me for this or that, and I don't want to be categorized this or that. I am stronger than the damages Dick and Pat left for me to exist with. I would not let Dick and Pat win, as if this really was a game, like I really was a willing participant eager to compete. The pain was sickening, the aches debilitating. I don't like this place I am at, not in any regard. This is sickening to me, and I am very disappointed with what Dick and Pat chose to do to me.

Regardless of how bad off I physically felt, it was necessary for me to "log roll" out and off of that hospital bed. It was time, the physicians said, "to try to walk." I don't precisely know how many days I was lying in that bed, but the best feeling I grew to embrace was *to just lie still*. It wasn't a time I was interested in journaling, so I cannot honestly recall which day I rolled, which day I began donning a gym suit, which day my friends came to attend to my personal needs. I am pretty certain "journaling" never entered my living field at that time nor for the upcoming days anyway! Nor months or some years onward!

I was in no mood to "offer my pain to the Lord for mercy."

This is how you know when the pain is almost impossible to bear: "Please don't take the catheter out. I am not going to feel that pain again of log rolling out of this bed." This is a clear indication to oneself and the world that a victim is in a substantial amount of pain. I am pretty sure pain medications did reduce some pain, but I was miserable. I was most comfortable lying down, not moving; however, the physicians were right. To avoid additional adverse medical situations, my body needed to start moving. It's time, it's imperative to begin moving all parts of my body. But…I didn't want to feel the pains. The introduction to the beginning of four months of Vicodin and OxyContin had largely begun. The four pelvic fractures, many fractured spinal processes on each side of my spine, my broken tailbone, whiplash (the cracking of a whip at thirty miles per hour, high-speed injury), broken ribs in addition to the road rash covering my entire body with sporadic gaping contusions, add in the punctured lung creating a difficulty to take breaths and hurting with each one of those breaths, I would eventually begin to walk, tears streaming down my face, and the healing was to begin. I remember the pain, and I cry. I feel the lingering chronic pain, and I cry.

Today is a very intriguing day. Obviously, this is years later than the times I just shared with you in the above-mentioned paragraph. I had a very nice visit with a neighbor about life today. Not the common surface talk to fill our time. This was a genuine loving conversation, taking a considerable amount of unhurried time, sharing a few areas of our lives with each other. Fellowship. Kind, considerate words, nods, and smiles. There were tears shed also, sharing memorable moments that were held deep in our hearts. After our spontaneous visit, I began to review my day that led up to these moments of a love-filled dialogue between two Christian women. I wanted to visit with her; she was kind to me. I felt loved in our communication, and I felt respected and cared about. *God is in our midst.*

This particular day, my morning prayers were not filled with demanding supplications for deliverance from the evil inhabitants and events in this world, nor the praying of the Psalms I have prayed for many years, which mimic my rehearsed prayers, as I have continued to beg the Lord for safety from evil, security in his protection—security, guidance, and refuge. Those prayers were on my heart but didn't take the precedence today which they normally do (and have for many, many years). No, the Holy Spirit wasn't shouting my name. Softly, I was led to seek out and pray Psalms of victory. By God's mercy and grace, I do recognize that God is in control and he is my Healer. Here is what is amazing: *my acceptance of his blessings occurred*. His peace, his joy, blessings—I accept them. Thank you, Lord. Surrendering is very important; I am in control of little to nothing. I surrender to you, Lord.

I have begun to accept God's healing and blessings upon me. He is transforming me into that unique, once very stubborn woman, who he has been working on for a very long time. How do I know? Because I feel it, I see it, I hear it. I am living it. I have accepted what he has been longing for me to accept, and today is a glorious day. This is the day the Lord has made. I will be glad, and I rejoice.

My back pains make me cringe, and I can hardly keep writing as my neck is very weak and I am in extreme discomfort. It's typical for me to write only for a very short period of time as there comes a time as I sit and write, I can't hold my head up any longer. I have only retyped a few lines, and I am just about done for this day. I write with tears because I want to finish this book to share with you so many truths, tragedies, and transformations. I want you to have information and guidance and awareness to have tools to confront evil and make a determination to do what is right no matter what you could and quite possibly lose.

I reiterate, do the right thing, always believe in yourself, and advocate for the truth in all things.

What I am trying to say is that God is blessing me. I receive and I accept those blessings. We cannot accept only the trials, the pains, the heartaches, and the judgments. We must recognize and receive what God is pouring out to us. Open your spirit to true acceptance and belief in God's gifts to us. I am not talking about worldly, tangible gifts such as money, innumerable possessions, and any other idol we long for secularly. I am speaking of the peace of God which passes all understanding, living, in word and in action, the promises that God will guard my heart and my mind in Christ Jesus. I have never felt what I have experienced today. God's peace is promised to guard those of us who pray—with thanksgiving—about everything. It's really not exciting for me to say, "Thank you, God, that Dick ran me down and dragged me for twenty-five feet and attempted to destroy me in every possible way." What I say to God is "Thank you for loving me, thank you for blessing me."

Today I experienced an inner calm. I have to say that it is something I have never experienced. I have an abundance of symptoms from many diagnoses, and it's common knowledge that all these symptoms in the combinations that are present cause extreme difficulty to successfully treat all or even some. It's been a whirlwind of treatment trials. It lasted for years, all sorts of treatments. I really can't believe I am saying this: I never believed this day would come! I feel God's peace, and it brings me to tears because I have explored many treatments, and nothing was beneficial to me to the extent that God's peace has provided to me. I am in amazement tonight. God is blessing me with genuine, almost-tangible peace even through the pains. The pains are often unbearable, and God's peace is present.

This peace, this calm, is not to say my day was filled with my ways. I am human and God gifted me with emotions to help me through the trials and tribulations, the accomplishments, and the many other events I experience. Today, I shed tears, I felt hurt, I felt slighted, I felt disrespected, I shed more tears. Still, today I am experiencing a supernatural peace.

I sat outside. In the stillness, the Holy Spirit covered me with peace and love, and yes, I did accept his healing, his joy, and his peace. Today is glorious.

"Getting up to walk" gave me a stark fright of the tragedy's repercussions as the blood pooled into my left thigh, suggesting a large hematoma. Information all unfamiliar and unbeknownst to me, I was continually being surprised with the many unexpected arrivals of pains and blood issues. That particular region of my body is changed. I am sure there was more than one occasion I demanded the presence of the surgeon in my room in the evening as I panicked with ongoing pains and unexpected happenings. It's now a site of enlargement, discoloration, and scarring—the second physical daily reminder to me of an evil tragedy that happened to me years ago. I am not a vain person, but no amount of toning and exercising heals the flesh and repairs it to its original state. It's a large and fatty fleshy part of my leg and is literally heavy to hold. The area of this hip and thigh is an area of numbness. That metal attachment on Dick's truck dug into my body from the rib area on down to my thigh. I had great providers to repair that which could be repaired. I am grateful. The evidence remains as a stark reminder that someone on God's created earth, a human being God created to worship him didn't want me alive. It's no one's right to take my life or to even attempt that feat. It's God's decision as to when my heart shall stop beating, not Dick's or Pat's. Many times when I have tried to simply sit still in gratitude to God for his blessings, invading thoughts and images vividly appear: which parts of Dick's truck's undercarriage entered, injured, and manipulated my body in the hundreds of places? These horrible intrusive thoughts crowd my peace and none of which have a place in my healing. I wonder if Dick will drive that truck again, and still, I wonder, is the productivity in his life at all interrupted by the past horrific memories as my daily being is constantly interrupted? Again, no place in my healing to picture these tragedies all over again.

Yesterday Dick was released into the general public, under the supervision of a parole officer obviously. Dick was sentenced to eighty years in prison; fifty years were suspended, and he served sixteen years. It's obvious the time assigned to serve is actually quite a bit more than the time that is actually served. It's very common for a perpetrator to serve a third or less of his/her sentence and then look forward to a soon upcoming release.

Approximately 480 days prior to the evil attack Dick placed upon me and subsequently succeeded at, he completed a typing/comp project which denoted his New Year's Resolutions—the first New Year's Resolution, *"To get a driver's license so I can do those horrible things people like to read about in the paper,"* assignment completed and turned into the assigning educator (forwarded to school administration ten days after the date on the assignment). I often wonder why an educator would wait ten days to hand in an assignment to administrators that spewed with threatening abnormal desires.

Check: swimmingly accomplished! Dick made nationwide news. His deliberate attempted homicide was plastered in newspapers and newsfeeds all over the country.

Additional resolutions he proudly denoted were the following: killing the tooth fairy, stop screaming at my answering machine, get a job so I can afford ammo, improve typing grade, taste human flesh, make a movie about Hitler, find out what really happened in *Roswell, New Mexico*, find out who really killed JFK, invite blood relatives to a barbecue, and lastly, shoot someone on a camping trip and say it was an accident. (Dick's original list is included in the addendum)

When Dick attempted to kill me, trying to "make good" on his number one resolution, he was maintaining a 0.86 GPA; I would find that very disconcerting, whether I was his parent or an educator. He was a sophomore in high school, a critical time in his life. Was there an IEP? No. Was special education considered? No. Reports indicate at one time in his life he was in gifted education. There simply was no interest by anyone to delve into Dick's life to assist him in doing the best he could in school. In the ensuing investigation, it loudly came to light (may I add, "a tad bit late" for the prevention of a hideous crime) that there were quite a few disconcerting circumstances that were literally hung, mismanaged, and wrongly unmanaged, such as Dick's parents not responding to the school personnel's letter suggesting that Dick attend "summer school." There was no response from the parents, and no further follow-up by the school personnel mimicking each entities indifference regarding Dick. Dick was falling through the cracks. I don't understand why the focus was to encourage the parents to entice Dick to attend summer school; a focus should have been on Dick to work on his grades during the school year, the time when his GPA was plummeting very quickly. The tragedy he inflicted upon me was reportedly not the beginning of his hardships. His hardships began many months, even years, possibly many years prior (evidence indicates his hardships possibly began around second grade, but only *once* was evaluated by a psychologist in all these years), when those who had contact with him in many regards tragically ignored him, pretended not to notice him, avoided him, outrightly shunned him, placated him, and the few who were intimidated by him were included in this vast assembly of people who made no efforts to ascertain even just a crumb of what it was that Dick needed and required to be healthy, whole, and successful in school and additionally, in his life. Dick was hurting in the life God gave him. It became clear that nobody wanted to help Dick. You get it; he was an outcast and vastly marginalized. He didn't play sports and wasn't given any attention. You and I both know that when a student thrives in sports and participates in extracurricular activities, the students, their parents, and other students involved in sports along with their families will associate and bond with educators and administrators of all sorts, continually establishing relationships. This isn't rocket science; this is reality in this culture.

This isn't profiling, we all will attest to this; this is school culture in America. Dick was screaming for help for all the years of his life, and no one took the essential life-giving time to assess his needs and determine exactly what it was that Dick needed to grow, to learn, to succeed, to feel healthy, and to be a productive part of a community.

There are many of you who do not live with the charity to help others; however, we all have a moral obligation to step up, put yourself aside, and help a child. Don't follow the culture of this world; be an image of Jesus Christ. Dick, a child, was screaming for help, at many times inaudibly. Dick's parent(s) met with school personnel upon his submission of his New Year's Resolution list. The New Year's Resolution list contents concerned the instructor, so days later (about ten), she shared the composition project with the school counselor(s) and with one of the assistant principals. Dick's parents met with the high school administration, a counselor. After that meeting, Mr. Awks, Dick's assigned counselor, decided immediately to discontinue giving his services to Dick, as there was a "conflict of interest." The reports indicate that Dick was fine with continuing counseling with Mr. Awks, but Mr. Awks was "troubled" by what he thought he heard Dick say, that Dick was going to bring a gun to school. Mr. Awks removed himself as Dick's counselor.

True. Sixteen years, I continue to shake my head and believe there was so much detriment caused by others' lack of interventions, which were, of course, outside of Dick's own abilities and personal responsibilities to seek growth and health. Waywardness by supposed mentors enveloped Dick everywhere he trod.

You will notice throughout this book the vagueness or lack of explanation of something that really is important to expound upon. Allow me to explain. There is very little written information about this student. This vague, under-reporting of a very serious situation involving a troubled student and the school administration which the community paid highly to succeed in their responsibilities, but in fact largely failed, is a disgrace and nefarious.

Dick's mother insisted and maintained that insistence, quickly convincing all responsible school personnel (those who are responsible and required to refer a student to a mental health evaluator, psychologist, or psychiatrist to duly obtain a thorough evaluation, an appropriate assessment, and accurate diagnoses) that the New Year's Resolution List does not in any way show that Dick is having any troubles. "He is just bored with his class contents." Conversing with school personnel, it was decided upon that since they all agreed that Dick was "just bored," they would try to make arrangements for him to take some classes that were more "fun." He was interested in culinary arts, information technology perhaps. My eyes are seriously rolling out of disgust for such lame intervention, an agreed-upon neglection, and abandonment of duties. Mr. Less, the school's principal (he did hold a counseling certificate), responded to Mr. Awk's self-removal from providing any service to Dick by stating that he would now begin to oversee Dick. Unfortunately for many, many people, Mr. Less never met with Dick or his parents or other personnel regarding Dick and his behaviors and success or lack of success in his studies. There was no further communication between Dick (nor his parents) and *any* school personnel. Dick's GPA plummeted to 0.83 (last GPA recorded). Are you slapping your palm against your forehead like I have for the past sixteen years? I would imagine some of you are.

School and police reports are very conflicting. It's *possible* Mr. Less did meet with Dick one time, or possibly, he never did. No further reporting was made. I may have mentioned earlier in this book that all reporting in the available information (I have seen every page of evidence) is confusing, inconsistent, and filled with incongruences. Not one individual in all the entities involved strove for truth and to do what it takes to have all questions answered in their entirety. Refusing to participate in conversations with media, administration keeps answers succinct: "I was taken off the case," "I cannot comment," and the most intriguing and words of lies and betrayals is this: "We did all we could."

Continual slaps in my face and in Dick's face. No justice in any regard, on any level, with any entity involved. Heartbreaking? Yes! Inexcusable? Without a doubt!

Mrs. Lacks (the teacher who assigned the composition of the New Year's Resolution list) divulged somewhere in this fatty confusion and unprecedented chaos that the room where she stored the discs that contained the New Year's Resolution's lists was at some point broken into. Dick's assignment disc had been removed, erased, and miscataloged into the disc holder; there was no investigation. *There is no police report* regarding this crime. Was someone covering up the fact that Dick's list was warranted for a police investigation or that Dick was screaming for help and potentially in need of a mental health evaluation, in which neither occurred nor was anything properly orchestrated by the appropriate authorities? Was it a student who broke into and burglarized the room where property was stored and tampered with? Was it Dick and his friend Pat who enjoy informational technology? Was it a cover-up by a teacher, counselor, principal, assistant principal or other school personnel, family, and friends? We will never know. An investigation was nonexistent, so obviously, there is no report. Burglary, tampering with evidence, these are crimes wherever they are committed. Someone, possibly several or many individuals, is/are living with this information which is still coming to the forefront of their conscience and will continue to do so for all time. Crimes were committed, no law enforcement officer completed a report. This immense lack of action, unanswered questions and carelessness, created an unprecedented hole. That's my opinion only. For those involved in any way imaginable, they are obviously content with where they have hidden all the questions left unanswered and the crimes unsolved. Many betrayals leave many disappointments. Their lack of involvement causes much confusion.

The disc is blank. There was no resolution. No one considered these events important. There are no timelines. This is extremely vague and unacceptable. Apparently, this activity was no big deal to anyone, not even to the assigned student resource officer.

Friends, cliques, associations, acquaintanceships, things actually can and will get swept under a rug rather quickly and stealthily.

In which school is a student permitted to don long black coats and exhibit the wearing of vampire teeth throughout the school day?

This is *inexcusable*.

In which school is a student allowed to make threats involving a gun and not be further investigated nor in any way held accountable? No investigation by a student resource officer and no investigation by a local police department. In which school would information as such not be expounded upon in a student's files if, in fact, such usage of words actually existed? How is a counseling session even conducted if the determination of the words used in the session is unidentifiable? Inconclusive endings are hanging and these dangling questions are unacceptable.

The assigned counselor *wasn't sure* what was "actually" uttered (this hired professional, whose responsibilities included counseling and guiding students, sought out no explanations nor any further communications to eventually evolve at the truth and subsequently come to a conclusion about what was uttered and why and so on).

This is *inexcusable*.

Which school allows counselors to simply drop their services because they don't like what a student says and no longer wants to meet with the student/parents, feeling intimidated but not contacting local police authorities to share the information regarding a gun?

This is *inexcusable*.

Which school allows *undated* chicken scratches of abbreviated ink adhered onto *adhesive* paper to be an official part of a student's *confidential* report/file?

This is *inexcusable*.

Which school allows a counselor to "drop" counseling services to a student and not be required to follow up with the particular administrator (in this particular case, a principal who held a counseling certificate) who offered and vowed to oversee the student's performance, to actually gain the knowledge to determine whether or not the troubled student is truly a recipient of necessary counseling and referrals if necessary?

This is *inexcusable*.

What principal would agree to oversee a student who is struggling and exhibiting undoubtably mental health hardships but will not invest the crucial time to actually counsel, guide, and direct or meet with the struggling student/parents to develop a relationship with them and subsequently assess the needs and determine if further evaluations are warranted, possibly referring and obtaining evaluations and assessments from community experts outside the school district?

This is *inexcusable.*

Who on a school board would allow school administrators and randomly involved personnel to ignore the knowledge of crimes then forego an appropriate thorough investigation of a burglary, tampering with evidence, destruction of the evidence, and the damage to property case?

This is *inexcusable.*

Which school does not have the affinity to enforce the responsibilities of the proclaimed qualified personnel to adhere to the mandates to ensure the testing and the evaluating of all the students, including the students who are severely failing academically, and putting in place a program to meet each student's needs for their individual success?

This is inexcusable.

Which school upholds the dismissing, ignoring, and allowance of complacency with regard to the requirements of duly conducting proper assessments to accurately determine the cause of failing grades, exhibition of inappropriate and bizarre behaviors, along with the socially unacceptable demeanors which will cause harm to oneself and others?

This is *inexcusable.*

Which school, accredited, will not take full responsibility for the mental health evaluations necessary for a student to acquire an IEP to be successful in the classroom?

I am confounded about the magnanimous lack of intercessions on many levels, by many "educators" (those individuals considered professional staff, hired to perform these duties) that would have benefitted this neglected suffering student.

This is *inexcusable.*

What parents wouldn't respond and act expediently and proportionately to a letter from their son's high school, suggesting that their son attend summer school?

This is *inexcusable.*

What parent would allow their child to drive their (or any!) vehicle, when being informed of a New Year's Resolution list, wherein the number one resolution is screaming "stop—danger"?

1. "Get a driver's license so I can do those horrible things people like to read about in the paper."

   With knowledge and evidence of the many indicators that this student was conveying to many, his battling of a mental illness, he *was never* evaluated, assessed or diagnosed; there was no intervention of any degree by parents nor school personnel.

This is *inexcusable.*

What parent wouldn't step up to get their child the obvious necessary educational attention, mental health care, and emotional health care when continually witnessing unhealthy behaviors in their child, both at home and at school, for months and possibly years?

The parents who blatantly reneged on their covenant made with their child that "*he would not drive until he was successful in bringing up his grades*" with his GPA plummeting from a 0.86, now a 0.83, *was miraculously allowed to drive.*

This is *inexcusable.*

What parent wouldn't demand an initial and thorough police investigation (by an impartial law enforcement agency) of a crime wherein their child is considered a possible suspect even if the school and/or district was against the investigation?

There is no police report, so it's probable "suspect" isn't the proper term.

This is *inexcusable.*

What parent wouldn't fight for their child's "today" and "future" by showing care and concern by getting involved with and demanding a reasonable thought-out plan executed by the school personnel for her son to become a responsible successful student?

This is *inexcusable.*

What parent grants their young child while strug-gling in every area of his life the unsupervised freedom to joyride with other young friends while enjoying a pornographic magazine, hunting down a woman to kill and rape? Where is a child's supervision?

This is *inexcusable.*

Small in comparison to the huge picture, but minimally, what parent wouldn't strongly intervene *in any way* in her young child's life to help raise his 0.83 GPA in all ways that she can?

Unfortunately for many innocent individuals, Dick was allowed to fall through the cracks. In his home, as well as in the school district he attended, his parents and many school personnel made a choice not to guide him or even interact with him. No one at the school displayed any sort of care or guidance. Parents, counselors, and the principal agreed in unison that "Dick was fine." *Common sense arises in me that all these red flags*: the unusual behaviors and the long chain of events involving Dick which were witnessed by many at home and in his high school, the drawings during class on his body and on his papers displaying a sought-after darkness, the discussions of nudity and crimes (the offering to Jane of five dollars to see her boobs while in the classroom), the wearing of the long dark-col-ored trench coats and donning dark sunglasses, the wearing of the vampire teeth throughout the school hallways, the GPA of 0.83, the mentioning (to a counselor assigned to Dick) of the fact that he (Dick) would bring a gun to school, the *uninvestigated* criminal acts of burglary, theft, destruction of information (on a disc which was kept under lock and key), the infantile and strange behaviors that Dick was exhibiting in his home (where he lived with his parents and a sister), and perhaps strange occurrences seen by many more witnesses, which most likely have been undisclosed, undiscovered, or unreported, many events that were indignantly ignored *were unheeded and culminated into a pure lack of moral judgment on many individuals' parts.*

For an undiscovered reason to this day, it's evident the answers aren't sought out nor obviously are transparencies important for the integrity of that community, sixteen years later, or perhaps it is a successful, diligently deliberated cover-up—no truths, no admissions.

All blamed Dick for his dumb stunts. It's not at all black-and-white, my readers. Dick was not dumb. Dick was sick, very sick, and all those proclaimed professionals who were in his presence for months and years allowed him further sickness and impending demise, encouraging perdition.

These school professionals literally avoided and intentionally ignored Dick. Dick, who was only a struggling teenager, whose screams for help were left all unanswered in all ways. That's a tragedy.

I have the utmost reason to believe that the inactions of those involved with Dick would never have believed their obvious dereliction would be a contribution to the culmination of an attempted deliberate homicide...by simply ignoring a student's mental health.

Many shirked their responsibilities, they escaped consequences, but there are a couple of them that I believe may be feeling some authentic guilt about their lack of sharing truths and rightfully admitting their inactions were a contributing factor to Dick's accomplished resolution.

It's clear, *many* people in all walks of life in that community failed in what they were required to do. Dick was betrayed. Clearly that staff and personnel could care less about Dick. They ignored his cries for help. Dick was suffering terribly.

I have been betrayed. Those people who let Dick down daily for months and years, who allowed him to travel downward to perdition, are responsible in part for his demise, a very large part. Ignoring and avoiding an ill student is reprehensible and simply irresponsible.

In addition, I hold them responsible for my victimhood.

When people do not take responsibility for what they have done that is wrong, they betray their own soul, they betray victims' souls.

Dick and I are victims, innocent victims, betrayed and suffering.

These uninvestigated crimes—however, the school district and their close associations most likely refer to them as events, incidences, occurrences, or unimportant matters, which were never even delved into by proper objective law enforcement authorities as a crime—have been ignored and closed. Closed and giving satisfaction to many, and for others, latched and cinched with no answers, no satisfactory explanations for those who believe it's deeper than it appears. The most likely panicky avenues to disregard the truth of something very real and dark left no one to be charged.

No police reports, no police investigations by an objective law enforcement agency, no outcomes. It's as if all this information is thrown into a deep dark hole for no one to retrieve. That's exactly where it's at: irretrievable in a deep dark place where some people have all the answers to all the questions that continually surround these months and years of tribulation.

There clearly was never effort to initiate a professional just investigation in an attempt to charge any individual(s) nor the desire to actually delve into a thorough objective investigation of the crimes within the school building (to rightfully bring to justice those who were involved). Disseminating as much as possible and eradicating the possible evidence of Dick's mental and emotional health issues, the many unanswered questions, *scream out loudly to me that this is a grand cover-up by many at the school and certain citizens in various professions within the city.* This clearly was a tragedy and pummeled forcefully into a near-fatal attack. Symptoms were left unattended to by many, and evil was encouraged to be spawned, yes, in the inactions of many.

Who would have thought that neglecting a student's loudly obvious mental health needs would eventually lead to an attempted deliberate homicide by the neglected student?

A red flag culminated into hundreds of red flags, which were all immorally unheeded.

If I haven't mentioned that these are strictly my own thoughts and opinions, let me iterate right now to you, these are my very own. It has taken me many years to be able to actually sit down and feel the excessive pain caused by the betrayal of so many people. I used to run from all this pain. Today I feel every bit of it. The feeling of these pains is necessary to heal, to bring closure, to accept that what I would have done in their shoes is not what they decided to do. Their ways are not my ways. The charity I have and share is not the desires of their hearts. To this day, I do not understand why the community publicly rallies around this principal, Mr. Less. They have comradery, they have cliques, associates who are all over rooting them on. Their life is fun and laughter; they support one another, even if it involves such darkness. Many citizens in that community showed their erroneous ways, which was giving their support to the darkness, the ignorance of truth.

Removing myself from that community, I have realized that the principal, Mr. Less, and all those thousands of former students he coached and loved out loud, were against me and have judged me (their unkind looks toward me and ignoring me surely signify their loyalty to the wrongs of the district and the administrators who failed Dick, took their toll, and encouraged me out of their community; they succeeded again, but not for the glory of God) for the filing of a civil lawsuit naming him and the district as defendants. I stand firm and do not agree with the wrongful antics by so many. I tried to unravel the evil. I didn't succeed on paper, but I am pretty certain that there are some Christian-involved parties that have repented for the darkness they were involved in. I did shine Christ's light and continue to do that which God commands.

Some school personnel decided to leave their posts, hopefully to begin to see that their goodness wasn't shining through, nor was their ill-cooperation acceptable in the darkness of that school district.

The principal had a lot of city/state/federal support as he was involved in education and sports in the areas for decades. No, I don't have a private investigator. I just read the newspapers and they reveal how great a man Mr. Less is considered and rallied around and how he taught, coached, and loved the students with exuberance. He seemed to gain notoriety in the state by his students, fellow coaches and fellow educators. He knew many people. For me, you already know how I feel about him. I would be the onlooker who would not emulate him nor support him in any regard. He took no responsibility in the care of Dick; in fact, his lack of any sort of assistance contributed to Dick's demise and subsequent atrocities. He absolutely did nothing to help Dick, maybe because Dick didn't play sports and there was no connection to the family. Dick and his family had no "association" with Mr. Less. They definitely weren't in the "in" crowd.

The newspaper stated how Mr. Less was arrested for a domestic assault, apparently a family member. An article on a later-dated paper says the charges were dismissed because a family member was the victim "wasn't hurt too badly and (she) wanted the charges dismissed." Turns out Mr. Less is a human and not a man to be worshipped. We have one God to worship and adore; it's Jesus Christ.

Back to the domestic family assault Mr. Less was taken to the jail for. The dismissal of charges? That move really confused me because it's a crime in Montana regardless if the "victim" asks for the charge to be dismissed. But there must have been some sort of association, again. Pondering who the judge was that dismissed this, was there again another connection of associations, acquaintance-ships, and cozy bonds.

It really is unfathomable to me and, quite frankly, seemingly sinful in many ways, that the behaviors of Dick were not sincerely and compe-tently evaluated by school personnel with a subse-quent mental health referral to a proper provider. Did this really happen? I continue to ask myself. Yes, sixteen years later! It's a question I place on myself many, many times.

So Dick's counselor dropped him like wildfire. The principal who offered to take on the "counsel-or's position" to guide Dick never met with Dick (there are incongruities—one place on a report it states they did meet; another writing entry states they never did meet). Dick was *never* referred to a mental health evaluator or a professional of any sort, *nor* was he ever initially evaluated by a school psychologist nor evaluated for an IEP. The crimes that were committed at the high school were never filed in a report made with the local police depart-ment. I don't know about you, but all this infor-mation, the incongruencies, the incompletions, and the inconsistencies truly shout that the truth has been hidden. Something truly is amiss. The truths are in a dark place.

The teacher who assigned Dick's New Year's Resolution list left the school district shortly after this ugliness unfolded (the wife of a former police officer).

You may think I have a disregard for law enforcement. I do not. Those who know me are aware that I breathe and bleed blue, but I do that only for the officers and police departments upholding the truths, thoroughness, and integrity. I have no place for departments that waver nor for those who do not seek answers, no matter who is involved—friends, associates—I seek truth.

I believe that many things are being hidden from the light. Maybe the light of many people, but it's not hidden from me.

Parents, teachers, educators, students, families, all of you deliberately choosing to read this book, listen to me. Allow my words to be your truths. It's our moral duty; it can literally mean life or death. We must pay attention to the things that are not common; in fact, what most of us would consider frightening, strange, unhealthy, absurd, and mind-boggling, call it what you will, label it as your professional supervisors deem appropriate, but if it's out of the norm, you as a citizen in a community need to show concern. If not for the individual's welfare displaying the unusual and dangerous behaviors, then act immediately for everyone else that could be affected, possibly maimed, or killed. You have a moral obligation to report a finding of concern to the appropriate authorities. You know what's right and what's wrong. You've participated in seminars, conferences, webcasts, etc. Don't allow yourself to be conformed to a culture that bullies you into doing things "their way." It's your duty as a citizen living in a community to act uprightly and strive to be honest and good. If your supervisor is against you giving truthful information to law enforcement, do it anyway. Learn to do the right thing regardless of how it may affect your selfishness of earthly dreams and earthly goals. Live selflessly for a perpetrator, a victim, a stranger. Your prompt and truthful reporting could mean you saving your own child's life. Yes, do the right thing. Be the person your children are proud to emulate. Be the person your child will be proud of. It's important to teach your children to do right; be just and be charitable. Your children are mimicking you. Do right.

School personnel and the parent(s) actually met and visited with one another on one occasion, or possibly two. The information available is very inconsistent. They shared their information among them: the strange behaviors, the infantile conduct Dick exhibited, the failing of courses in school, guns, burglary, property damage, and theft that occurred. Hundreds of students had much firsthand knowledge of Dick's words and behaviors for days, months, and years; they all walked together and passed one another in the same hallways. Some would receive notes from Dick, such as asking to see another student's breasts—yes, right there, in the classroom. He was going to pay a young girl to show him her breasts.

Readers, encourage your children to report abhorrent behaviors. If they are uncomfortable, accompany your child to report unwelcomed unsound events.

All in the school saw how he dressed and how he walked the hallways. Everyone could see the draconic drawings plastered all over Dick's large forearms. He was infatuated with the conversations of criminal behavior and darkness. He shared with his friends in school the crimes he desired to partake in. He point-blank asked others to join in on his desired plans to commit crimes. None of that information Dick shared over much time with his classmates ever made it to the administrators' offices, not even to the teachers in the classes these hoped for crimes were discussed. Not until after he ran me down did the information begin to be shared; it poured out; it fell out, mire and muck.

If the school your child attends does not offer a safe place to learn, the effects will eventually emerge. Be vigilant; be proactive with your child's success in the school building. Do all you can to protect your child. Commit to assisting your school district's promise of anonymity to safeguard your family as safe-reporting is essential if your child is in any way compromised in the classroom.

On May 23, 2003, in the midmorning class where art was being instructed, Dick told Dave that he wanted to kill someone. He told Dave that he wanted to rob a bank. Dave admitted to the police (who were investigating the attempted deliberate homicide I was victim to, on May 27, 2003, at 8:46 p.m.) that he and Dick have been having this type of conversation for two weeks. Dave spoke to the police about the pentagram and satanic symbols on Dick's arms.

Readers, it's imperative you teach your children to report danger even if uncertain if it will be carried out. Encourage your child to share the information with proper authorities.

Two weeks—readers, according to Dick's classmates, some of these conversations were held two and a half weeks before Dick tried to kill and sexually assault my corpse. Some reports indicate similar conversations had been held days and possibly only hours prior to the near-fatal strike. Encourage your child to not keep important information hidden. It could be your child's body in the ER. It could be you. Do what it takes to keep yourself and your children aware.

Police Reporting Information
(After the Crime)

A counselor hands a PAR report to the police officer investigating the ADH and, obviously in a state of defense, says to the officers that she "wasn't familiar with Dick." However, she later tells the police officer that Dave reported to her that he heard Dick state he wanted to kill someone. I don't know about you, but this language I attempt to interpret is not concise. This information which was part of the investigation is not concrete; it does not tell you if what Dick stated was on the day he tried to kill me or if it was after the crime that Dave reported the information to this counselor. Here's what I am saying: this information is not clear, this information is not dated, this is a mess of confusion that *has never had a clean finish*—inconclusive, poorly written, inconsistencies, stymied, no closure. All is unacceptable.

There are times that an outside impartial law enforcement agency is required to obtain absolute truth.

All of our schools must provide all students and personnel a safe place in which to report anonymously incidences that must be evaluated and investigated. All information must be confidential, and the reporter's name held in confidence. It's imperative that the reports are *dated* and filed properly. I would think that all reports would be mandated dated! It's imperative that all that is shared is dutifully recorded, to be placed into a file, correctly dated. No chicken scratch on scrap papers with adhesive, undated, and with no person's signage *allowed!*

This isn't elementary. This is unacceptable administration. Lack of thoroughness and a sharp lack of integrity was continually displayed. There were no consequences for the ongoing ambiguities.

Reporting to a Safe Place

Professionals are called to fastidiously record *all* information shared—no negating, no chastising, no berating of students allowed. Educators must be nonjudgmental and have and show compassion. If a student is an athlete or not, a band member, a language enthusiast or not, a theater/dance performer, black, brown, yellow, or white, an A student or not an A student, middle-class offspring or poverty-stricken, children of administrators and educators, children marginalized by some, regardless, educators are not afforded a right to delineate interventions. *We are all equal, and everyone deserves identical assistance for our welfare and must receive the best parts of our mentors' examples without discrimination.*

It's imperative, when all those choosing to work in the education field make a huge decision to guide, instruct, and lead students, that their performance in protecting all students, associating with all students, and leading all students, is in the students' *best interests*. All these professionals have a duty, and if they do not want to follow through with that duty and treat all students alike, abide by their professed responsibilities, then it's necessary for them to leave their post. It's not their decision to choose to assist some students and not others. They shall not be discriminatory. It's important that educators in all departments of the high school lead by example and do their best to make leaders of all students without a fee.

A Parent's Responsibility

It's not your student's educators', counselors', and principal's responsibility to raise your child; however, they have required obligations (regarding your child's safety in all realms) to adhere to in the presence of your child, as they promise to be healthy leaders, giving the guidance to protect your child's welfare while in their presence (body, mind, and soul). As you voluntarily take on the role of mother and father, and all responsibilities therein, you are required to raise your child with common sense, morals, love, respect, and an open door to allow your child to share all things. It's imperative, moms and dads and guardians, to continually teach your children to share with you or another trusted adult *anything* that is disconcerting, *anything* they question, *anything* they care or want to talk about. Open your ears, give your children your time, and listen to what they are *trying* to tell you. Watch them closely. Put your cell phones down, let the dishes wait for another hour, turn the television and radio off, and *listen to your children*. Do more than hear; listen to your children. Sometimes their efforts and pleas for you to finally listen will be in their inaudible efforts. Maybe they are terrified to talk to you. Maybe you don't invite them to share what's really going on in their school because you're too busy talking to your friend on the phone. Help your child to feel loved, valued, and cared about. It's in the most vulnerable moments a child will share information that you need to hear, information that he needs you to hear. Your actions will save lives. You taking some necessary time for your child to talk could be saving your child's life, your life, or a neighbor in your cul-de-sac. Delay no longer in living the way that you know is the right way, the way you should be parenting, today, *now*. Listen to your child. Love your child enough to listen. It's like pushing your baby in a stroller while talking to a friend on the phone. That is selfish, ludicrous behavior. Listen to your child when he is doing his homework; be with him. Save your family.

Slowly, every step deliberate with vastness, he walked the hallways of a large crowded high school, exuding confidently his towering stature at six feet, three inches. This soaring presence united with 250 pounds of mass, demanded a presence, in some cases, an audience, without effort. There was no mistake, Dick was always noticeable, but especially when he was wearing his vampire teeth, donning his large dark garments, and proudly wearing his darkened sunglasses. Yes, no typing error, he wore vampire teeth at the school. Apparently, that is permissible in that district.

When a child is ignored, when boundaries are not required, a child will feel and act like he can do whatever he wants without consequences. He wore what he wanted, appropriate or not, for the school district. He received no chastisement or reminders of the acceptable attire or accessories for this school district.

No love, no boundaries, no support quickly leads to immorality, danger, and darkness. A presence of being the god of oneself, falsely believing he has control of all things.

His loud, dark presence is radical and a figure that is largely impossible to be missed (ignored).

One would have to deliberately turn the head, turn the body, fidget aggressively and desperately in all one's power to remove oneself from his path. Red flags cannot be judged, large or small or medium; a red flag must be addressed. These are the exploits that require professional staff's attention. These are the opportunities an employee in education must take to show leadership and convey a direction understandable to the student to make aware, teach, and guide students to appropriate behaviors, dress codes, and how to behave with courtesy. Educators' leadership (without a fee) is required in all areas of education whenever you are guiding a student (someone's precious child). These are the instances where an educator must run toward a student who needs guidance and a lesson in boundaries. It is most definitely immoral to ignore this student and, worse yet, to deliberately *avoid* someone's child.

I am quite certain that staff of all departments are deemed competent to train and instructed when to take action. I am positive that education personnel are not instructed to ignore and avoid, on any occasion, regarding any student. Unfortunately, those high standards of care to be utilized and lived in the school were not adhered to for these particular red flags mentioned here involving Dick (someone's child). Those who take on the role of guiding students must always care enough to be nondiscriminating while appropriately assessing and addressing the plans necessary to assist a student in participating and succeeding in his school lessons.

These are the first undeniable red flags: flaunting his unique presence, confidently sharing his zest for darkness, and exuding large, living, long strides through the hallways of a crowded high school with hundreds of students in attendance, an incredibly large administration staff, and unending additional personnel. These undeniably noticeable demanders are unequivocally loud and most certainly demanding of everyone's attention—immediate attention. Missing, ignoring, avoiding, these inactions are the initial contributing factors that would eventually lead to an unforgettable tragedy—a preventable detrimental crime. These loud red flags were not heeded, in any regard.

I feel so much pain for Dick as I can imagine the sadness and abandonment he continually felt as he was being ignored and avoided by so many people, so many friends, families, and proclaimed educators. Dick was very ill, and my heart breaks for Dick.

Dick wasn't gradually slipping further into the deep darkness of evil thoughts and desires; he was plummeting into a world of fantasies of perdition wherein he was just about ready to check off his number one resolution on his New Year's Resolution list assignment. Recall, it was about 480 days before the coming of deep dread that he spent a few minutes with his mother in the counselor's office. He was left in charge to navigate the planning of his resolutions. So what? A couple of adults give him a few minutes of their time to tell him they aren't happy with his resolutions list, but "we will work together to help you get into some classes that are fun." Give me a break! School isn't about fun. It's about receiving an education that will help you to be successful and productive in society. Instead, the prison guards were his mentors for sixteen years. He became incarcerated as a child.

Interrupt red flags. Stand up and do the work you committed yourself to as hired professionals.

Teachers, you spend much of your days with people's children, hoping students model your behaviors. Be a moral model. Interrupt their wrong behaviors the first time you notice.

He had been on this path for a long time. It's obvious nobody cared enough to interrupt this darkness. No one had time for Dick; they were all too busy honoring and glorifying their own idols even though they signed up to mentor students. It's clearly undeniable that *someone* knew Dick was troubled. This is not a secret. Why would anyone ignore a sickness in a child?

He was not a popular student at the school. His parents did not have a seat of the "in-groups." As you could likely imagine, it became very apparent to Dick that absolutely no one cared enough to intervene in what they were watching him do every day. He was exerting himself to get noticed, to get some attention. He spent a minimum of eight hours in that school. "Why isn't anyone noticing me? I'll try something else" he would think as he desperately was needing, wanting, and begging for someone's attention and time. No avail yet.

You and I both know that we are all in need of love, of another's time and attention, to be recipients of encouragement and support. If we don't receive the basics of what is necessary for human survival, you know where that desolation can lead some people.

Hundreds of individuals noticed him. How could you not? One would have to make every extreme effort to do whatever possible to avoid his presence. He sauntered through the hallways now exuding a confidence, anticipating the next class where he would hopefully see his classmate's breasts for only five dollars.

No matter the continual darkening of and during his large presence and the months of proclaimed intimidating unknowns, no teachers, counselors, principals, assistant principals, paraprofessionals, lunch personnel, librarians, custodians, or ITs and no, no classmates, and not even his pal Pat of eight years ("eight" years of friendship; they must have shared a lot throughout these years, intimately getting to know each other on many different levels, without a doubt knowing each other very, very well), the friend who accompanied Dick on that tragic evening professed "joyride," *took a very important moment, would-be changing moment, to interrupt the ensuing darkness that was constantly surrounding Dick, the school, and the community.*

Make some plans as to how you will successfully interrupt potential danger. This is not a "wait to see if something like this happens again" moment. You must be prepared and must share your preparation with others. This is not something to take lightly. When you ignore potential danger, you are putting others' lives at a very high risk, possibly your child. Whatever your vocation, take it seriously.

Parents, *encourage your child to share information. It may save them or another.*

Educators, *be in the know of dangerous behavior in your school, whether the student is in a class of yours or not, whether you "know" him or not, whether you like him or not—this isn't a time to be judgmental.*

Administrators, *take your duties seriously and always do the right thing.*

Students, *report abhorrent, unusual, dangerous, repulsive, disturbing words and behaviors.*

Share what is observed, read, and seen.

I realize that I didn't mention anywhere yet the role the school psychologist played in this entire scenario. The school psychologist also was one who did not make an effort to interrupt these strange, distracting, and troubling behaviors that rang through the hallways of the high school. *No school psychologist was ever contacted to assist with Dick's ongoing* behaviors and failings—these behaviors that must not be permitted under any circumstances, behaviors and choices that must be addressed in a timely fashion but were incorrectly and almost fatally not addressed at all, ever. To be honest, I don't know if that high school had a school psychologist on-site, but what I do know is that *Dick was never referred to have an appointment with a school psychologist nor an evaluation with a provided school psychologist. He was also not referred off-site for a necessary evaluation and subsequent treatment. This entire situation minimally required further proper evaluation, thorough investigation on many levels with various agencies, and a final resolution that in many instances required total clarity and unambiguous answers.*

"School psychologist" isn't mentioned in the chicken scratching, the pupil report, nor the many police reports, nor the timeline created by law enforcement. *It's obvious that a school psychologist was never contacted, services utilized, nor a part of the initial unfolding and the end result of* these unheeded red flags. As you can see, it's really not an important topic to include because the fact is that a school psychologist, unfortunately, had no place in Dick's life. This decision of the administration to not allow a school psychologist to evaluate, assess, and diagnose Dick's ailments is not simply mind-boggling. This eradicate decision was reprehensible in many areas and certainly an irresponsible decision. A fault that demanded consequences, but consequences that never evolved. The knowledge of a school psychologist and the utilization of that personnel's services performed *really* should have been a huge part of this book. As things were turning dark and evil, the required inclusion of a school psychologist or a psychologist, psychiatrist, or perhaps a primary care provider *would have, with no doubt, changed all things*, most importantly rescued Dick from a hellish existence and subsequently hindered the attempted deliberate homicide (and the many, many "events" inside those bookends).

The expert's sought-after thorough assessment and appropriate mandatory treatment would have made a difference in so many ways, in so many lives…that I believe.

It's highly likely that including a *school psychologist* in Dick's school experience at the high school, or minimally referring Dick to a *primary care physician* to begin evaluations, would have interrupted, deterred, and possibly totally disrupted Dick's number 1 resolution attempt.

Dick's mother discussed displeasure with an assigned counselor. She carried on that the (astonishingly dark and evil) composition assignment Dick turned in to the teacher was "taken too seriously." That statement continues to leave me raw.

The written information collected during the criminal investigation from the high school is utterly astounding and screams of unacceptable, unfinished, inconsistent, and incongruent practices, created by many educators and administrators in the school district. All this obscurity demanded the supervision of another entity, an entity which upholds integrity.

These wide fields of inconsistent terms and statements that I have read over time and time again (as they rot in a file I hold in the den) over sixteen years continue to bombard me to the obvious fact indicating an incoherence, inharmonious and a subsequent clearly erroneous, hasty decision made by a judge making the ruling to dismiss the civil lawsuit I filed against the school district regarding their irresponsible near-fatal decisions *to refuse to intervene and error magnanimously* in the still small light (obviously seemingly to the administration) of Dick's continual disturbing darkness. A school district's subjective rendition of this immensely evil unfolding of a resolution was to not act upon the red (scarlet) flags: inaction, ignoring, slighting, avoiding, scapegoating, defensiveness, deciding not to live rightly with responsibility. Dick's unending trails of red flags were loudly deemed "inconsequential" and loudly deemed as unnecessary to be addressed.

The crimes of burglary, tampering, destruction of property, damage to property, as I mentioned previously, *were never reported to the local police department*. There are no police reports. This fact in itself is horrifying. Who gets to determine when an actual crime is reported, and who determines when it is satisfactory to just keep all involved silent? These crimes had perpetrators, unknown how many, but no investigations were ordered, sans no charges. That's distasteful and simply immoral. My thoughts, my words, someone was acting in a wrongful position to cover this all up. I feel this, I believe, and I stand solid on my beliefs.

Mind you, these are all (uninvestigated, unaddressed) components in plain sight, leading up to an attempted deliberate homicide. These cover-ups (to the burglary, tampering crimes, etc.) move toward the covering up of all the atrocities committed by the district's personnel in trying to cover up all that transpired regarding Dick. This is pure chaos and unacceptable.

Be mindful; all the information I have revealed reportedly came to light to the police *after I was run down by Dick and Pat.* (That's the information I have received and what I and the entire world have been led to believe.) Do I know the truth? No. There are so many unanswered questions in so many areas regarding the school district and its non-reporting of incidences that indicate to me a high disregard for integrity.

The cover-ups, the lack of truthful information, the total lack of any investigations whatsoever are the refuse which were used by a judge to dismiss a civil lawsuit naming the school district and Mr. Less as defendants, along with Dick's parents, and the prior decision to dismiss Pat, the passenger, from any liability.

A thorough investigation of the neglect and the many, many misdeeds and inactions performed by the school district's personnel was inarguably warranted—warranted to be investigated by an "outside" law enforcement agency unaffiliated with this city. There were too many close relationships, acquaintanceships, associations, friendships, comraderies, mentorships, alliances, dealings, memberships, etc., among the police, the school district personnel, and the judge for an impartial investigation to be completed and for rulings to be made with complete justice. An objective investigation would have led to appropriate charges and fair rulings. Too much intimacy in the governing agencies involved, using their leverages in various ways, made it *impossible* for perpetrators to be sought out, named, and charged, rulings to be fair and just, and a victim to be served honestly with justice.

With all the inconsistencies, unexplained crimes, inconclusive words and statements, and undefined jargon, all is unmeasurable and *impossible to clearly rule justly*.

Words thrown about on paper, scribbled without names, dates, signage, explanation—a thorough investigation would reveal much; however, in this "type" of environment (intimate and close-knit), even that was not afforded the victim(s).

> *Displeasure*
> *"Had it in for..."*
> *Accused*
> *Implying*
> *"Could not retrieve..."*
> *Erased*
> *She thought*
> *May have been*
> *Noticed*
> *"Money offered to see her boobs"*

And these are words from *one* page of information regarding the investigation of the *criminal act* Dick perpetrated—all undone, no investigative reporting.

It's unnecessary to fill my book with words and statements that shout out loudly of *inconsistencies*. Yes, I am disappointed with the large lack of truth and justice, disgusted by the continual lack of interest, concern, and follow-through to even begin to complete any equation.

Dick's mother and the involved administration vowing to oversee Dick in the school setting all believed that working together to get Dick into some "fun" classes would be the answer to his boredom (mental illness, darkness, and evil).

This is for real, my interested readers. What? None of this can be made up. I have all the information in my home. These are not lies. I shake my head along with you. This makes no sense to me. This is ludicrous, erroring in so many ways on so many levels involving so many individuals, and I pray to God that this sort of months and years of mishandling of serious issues will not again prevail in any school. This is an outright dereliction of many, many people's duties.

There absolutely cannot be a just decision when the *governing of secrets* in the various levels of the relationships of all involved in the suit are paramount in one's life. There can be no justice when there is no objectivity. People who are ruled by their own idols will not seek what is right and just; it's not important to them. There must be a recusal of self if one *cannot* judge fairly, whether it is her conflicts within herself that will prevent her from judging fairly or the conflicts outside of herself that promote her injustice; she should not have been allowed the judgeship on my lawsuit.

I often wonder why another judge recused himself and this ruling judge went full speed ahead like a freight train without contemplation but with intention to protect others, and who had the responsibility to mentor her and to remind her of taking an inventory to determine if that self she lives truly can be impartial? Were checks and balances to determine objectivity reviewed?

Can a judge under oath be impartial when her daughter(s) has participated on the same sports team with one of the school administrator's daughter? This isn't a "miniscule" nor an "inconsequential" association; this is years of associations.

Regarding the crimes committed within the school building prior to the attempted deliberate homicide and the information utilized to make a ruling on the civil lawsuit, let me share my feeling and my thoughts. Magnanimous ill-willed decisions were made with the following in mind: cliques, friendships, promises, expectations, cover-all bottoms, secrets, lack of follow-through, allegiances, lack of follow-up, lack of necessary referrals, lack of dated reports, lack of signed reports, lack of thorough evaluations and investigations, a bold string of absences and incongruencies, checks and balances not maintained, unfairness, and what I call, criminally, a judge sought to nullify all truths and instead sought injustices. For what reasons? Benefitting who?

Can a judge truly be impartial as her husband maintains a membership of an organization (encouraging juniors in high school to strive for leadership for a fee) that works *closely* with this particular district's high school's counselors and principals?

I call smelt.

Intermingling, webbing, indisputably no possibility of justice.

It's no secret the judge and her husband are alumni of this particular high school, pointed at in the lawsuit, naming Mr. Less, the principal for many years there, as a defendant. Their daughters excelled not only in academics but sports, and that principal presiding over that school was loved. All rallied around as he participated in the athletes' activities. The judge and her husband held a deep loyalty to that school, the entire school district.

Be real and admit along with me that *academically and collegiately involved children + involved parents = associations, acquaintances, friendships, loyalty, shared information, expectations, leagues of* their *own,* even signing the same campaign ad (with very few names), shouting out integrated support to her friend. This isn't coincidence; these are facts that when your daughters are involved in sports and amazing academia, you are going to be somewhat intimate with their mentors (educators, counselors, principals, assistant principals, coaches). This isn't rocket science; this is life, and it's loud.

Too many associations on many different levels among the judge, her family, the police department, and the school district's personnel shouts to me there is huge "subjectivity" involved.

There is absolutely no way that this judge would be able to judge fairly with all of her and her husband's associates rallying and rooting together for their beloved favorite high school whose daughters shared the same team name.

In severe pain, I sat on a bench in courtroom number 2, and you, Judge Black, having charge over this lawsuit, came sauntering in with your hair all a mess and your wrinkled black robe all twisted, your black glasses unleveled on the bridge of your nose, as if you just crawled out of bed. Your red stilettos stomping onto that hard-tiled floor with no hose, and you looked at me with a strange expression (as if I was representing all the wrongdoers), and you said, *"Unforeseeable, case dismissed." You looked coldly toward me and that engineer in you was going to put me in my place. I found that very strange. But I was too close to so much garbage going on with the criminal act and the civil suit that I was blindsided to the truth, and it took me sixteen years to even want to sit down and take a look at your relationships to those who were actually in the wrong regarding much. It's obvious your relationships with so many of these people trumped justice, and that sickens me.*

I have even run across a wedding announcement wherein a man who shared your married name was marrying a woman whose surname was that of an assistant principal at the high school. I am thinking that there were many, many associations. Most all of you involved in these events have lineage in the community for many years and have acquaintanceships of many kinds on many levels, and that would make it impossible for you to rule justly. I didn't know sixteen years ago how deep this all went. "Who you know" can be a type of lifestyle which may work for some people, but it's always immoral for anyone to participate in. I choose life—a life that is fair and just.

I did run across an article in which you resigned your judgeship quite early in your career, which surprised me because you were going gang-busters with your boldness in the newspapers. The newspapers report that you were a victim in a slip and fall case at a famous venue. I would deem that "unforeseeable," as you wrongly judged my suit, but you reaped much from that entity you sued. Sometimes I just don't understand how inequity reaps, but money doesn't heal and money doesn't get us to heaven.

You decided that no one (school district, Dick's parents, Dick's passenger, Pat) will be deemed responsible for all the neglect and failings they contributed to where Dick was involved. I disagree with your rulings, dismissals. Those named as defendants in the lawsuit failed miserably; they failed Dick and many others of us in the ripples of abandonment. You set, instead, a precedence in the state of Montana, quite possibly throughout the nation as the many events and rulings were shared all over the United States of America, maintaining that all involved in the raising and the education can succeed in their professions when ignoring the *obviate mental illness overtaking this young student.* This is immorality.

First and foremost, however, you and I worked for the same county. You shared your disregard for me many years prior to presiding over this lawsuit I filed. *You in no way had any business choosing to preside.* You had an obligation to recuse yourself as for many years you disliked me and showed that to me.

It's evident that many were failed by all those who rejected the welfare of Dick; that rejection, deliberate rejection, initiated tragedy. Where some counselors desire to mentor, others choose to run away, failing the student in many ways and, in turn, failing many others in his dust.

I try to keep this book concise. I try my best to not be distracted by strong feelings and thoughts. You must understand, I suffer much from a traumatic brain injury, and my brain will never again function as an uninjured brain. Please bear with me as I attempt to sort this out for you so it is clear to you.

A "gun" was brought up in a meeting with Dick's parent(s) and other school personnel. I use a parenthesis often because I don't want to exclude someone that may have attended this meeting. The reports differ, filled with inconsistencies, but I want to include someone because I don't want to write erroneously. Anyway, this information was never reported to the local police department. *If* this information was given to the high school's school resource officer, she obviously neglected her duties in many ways as this information was never brought to the attention (using an official report) of the main law enforcement agency in this area. There was plenty of time to turn in this pertinent information to the police department. Dick floundered on his own accord with his own agenda for many months without receiving an essential assessment and intervention. Dick actually was giving the school district and the police department much opportunity to come to the reality that there was much to attend to. Dick fell further downward into the darkness, and the principal who offered, elected, and agreed to take on and oversee Dick as a counselee never met with Dick or his parents or educators of Dick. Dick's behaviors and performance in school were never again assessed after the visit about the list. The negligence of the school staff and many personnel is clearly evident in many instances, on many levels, and in wretched regard. Dick was left unchecked and succeeded in completing his number 1 New Year's Resolution because as noted on a note in the counselors' office, "no one took any of Dick's words, idiosyncrasies, demeanor, and behaviors *seriously*." Just as his mother, an LPN conveyed, the school district's personnel's lack of action chimed right in with her that they all believed Dick was "fine." Dick was not fine and that was clear.

The school district's administration allowed Dick to further deepen his road to a perdition, an ugly demise. Dick received no assistance from any staff, no intervention for additional counseling, no referral to a therapist, no referral to a school psychologist, no referral to a primary care physician, no referral to a community psychologist or a psychiatrist. Not even a general health examination was performed on Dick which would in fact have indicated to the primary care provider that the exhibitions of Dick's behaviors should be referred to the experts in the field of psychiatry. There simply was no guidance given in any area. The counselor dropped him, the principal dropped him, didn't even attempt to meet with him for that matter, and Dick was left to deal with what was diagnosed months after the attack as a perpetual psychosis—a deteriorating psychosis is what the report says here, a disease that was continually worsening. These debilitating diagnoses are provided by two experts in the field of psychology/psychiatry.

It didn't matter to anyone that Dick walked the high school halls in gothic apparel and dark sunglasses; apparently it was permitted in that school district. I don't think it was, but with inaction by so many people, either it was permitted or the ones in authority overseeing the students didn't care what Dick did—no boundaries, no support.

Not only was Dick failed by teachers, parapro-fessionals, counselors, a principal, assistant princi-pals, his friends and classmates, students, their fam-ilies; myself and my friends and family were also failed. I would have to say that a community was failed. We expect leadership and mentoring from those requesting to be a part of the team of educa-tors, and we deserve an expertise in their responsi-bilities and the expectation of moral standards to guide the community's children. There prevailed a damning list of inactions. Mandatory actions were required to be taken by the school district's per-sonnel. They did fail a community, the society that trusted in their promises to do the best that they can for the welfare of students and families.

Students must not be "left behind" in math and reading, nor shall they be left behind when suf-fering a mental illness.

Tragic, sinful, and immoral, *none* of the indi-viduals (and *there are* many) who were aware of the events in this disturbing scenario that went on for many months before the near-fatal strike will admit any knowledge of the circumstances. A counselor who had access to Dick's records stated in a police report she didn't know anything about Dick; she wasn't "familiar" with Dick. I pray to God that from that point forward, if any stu-dent exhibited failing grades, potential threats, restricted dress, intimidating demeanors, strange behaviors (warranting investigation), disregard for school personnel and property, this student's counselor will intervene timely and appropriately and accurately denote times, dates, names, etc. It really should be mandatory when information is gained about a student that could be problematic and dangerous, that this same information is shared with all administration. As I reread my entries, I shake my head. This sounds elementary, but it's true. All I reveal is true. Neglectful and sinful are the terms I use to encompass many errors.

Intervening must be mandatory. Outrightly interrupting the dangerous resolutions that have been broadcast to the school must be mandatory.

If you are a counselor and you are intimidated by the word "gun" used by a counselee, you better give up your post. If you remain at your post, it's your duty to get the actual facts and determine what it is that is transpiring. Get the *accurate* information to determine what it is that is transpiring. Gain clarity and congruency and do what you signed on to do: mentor and guide. Dig in and help, encourage, and support those who are being left behind.

If you don't want to obtain the facts, it's time for you to resign your post, but prior to that, make sure your local police department is aware of a student threatening to bring a gun to school.

Most importantly, for the safety of all, I pray that students' parents begin to take strange behaviors exhibited in the home very seriously and do all that it takes to get the necessary intervention to help their child with mental health issues. Let us remind our children, as students in school, *be aware* of another student's behaviors and their cries for help. Sometimes it's important to take our minds off of ourselves and be selfless on occasion; they, too, can help to prevent *unnecessary tragedies*.

None of the individuals who counseled Dick, who taught Dick, paid to mentor and guide Dick, who was in Dick's life on a daily basis (at home and at school) were held accountable for his tragic demise, nor will they with plain decency and humility (promised integrity to protect students) admit any wrongdoing. These individuals, so innumerable, deliberately ignored all *red flags* exhibited by Dick for months, turns out, actually for years. If in fact, those mentoring and guiding at the school were fearful, a law enforcement agency should have been contacted. That's rudimentary. Ignoring red flags encouraged the defendant's waywardness. Nobody cared how he behaved, the disgusting words he shared with his classmates. He was in charge, and he showed us just how in charge he was. The school district's turning a blind eye made him all the more invincible.

They pretended he wasn't there, deliberately not noticing him, and then...he obtained attention from all over the United States of America.

Parents have a moral responsibility to attend to a child's mental, emotional, physical, spiritual, and social welfare. If your teenager begins to display atypical behaviors—for example, storing one's own urine in a bedroom for six months, sleeping at the bottom of a parent's bed, demanding that a light be left on during the night, maintaining that he controls the weather and additionally has the symbols written for you to see—it's your parental responsibility to get your child some help. It is paramount to lifesaving that any disturbing behavior be addressed with the appropriate experts. This is a parent's responsibility. If you as a parent are aware of these abnormal behaviors, you have a moral responsibility to your child, your family, students, and society to obtain the necessary treatment for your child to live healthfully in a community.

Living a life of disturbing behaviors out loud, out in the open, in a closed room, inaudible, all warrant an intervention. Dick's family failed him. Again, many more professed adults chose to lie and repeat, "He's fine." I refute all their words, "No, it was very obvious for a long time that Dick was not fine."

Dick's mother walked quickly and nervously around the courtroom floors, eyeing me up and down as we await for a judge to preside at the sentencing hearing, holding tightly onto her rosary beads. She looked at me with scorn. What?

Readers, have you ever read *This Present Darkness*?

I feel like this community definitely is a setting in one of the chapters of the book I mentioned. Evil is real, it is here, and I was in the midst of Satan and his angels as St. Michael fought on for God's glory.

I hate the evil that surrounded me. It disappoints me when I return to that chapter in my life, and I am cognizant of the dishonesty and ruthlessness displayed by so many. The sin of pride is among the worst I experienced. I, too, am a sinner, just like the rest of the people God created. I repent and I forgive all the people who chose evil over good, doing so for many, many reasons. Even the judge who tried to convince me, she could rule objectively. I forgive her. Fairness was not present.

The red flags were becoming more and more scarlet...and were continually being unheeded.

Dick's mother and father attested to how their son, at sixteen years of age, slept at the bottom of their bed, how he stored his own urine in his bedroom for six months. As a parent, wouldn't that be disconcerting? Wouldn't a responsible parent have that child examined by an expert in mental/behavioral health? His parents emphatically failed Dick, continuing to say that "he is fine."

Those are just a couple of the disturbing behaviors of a sixteen-year-old that were categorized as behaviors that were "fine." Dick was living a life filled with mental and behavioral illnesses and all adults in his world left him to continue in his downward spiral. No teacher, no counselor, no principal, no assistant principal, no paraprofessional, no school nurse, no guardian, no school psychologist (oh, that's right, I remind myself, he never was evaluated by a school psychologist) referred Dick to proper health/medical care nor to proper authorities. Dick suffered with constant dangerous and ill health which placed himself and society in great danger.

Struggling, exhibiting unhealthy behaviors in his daily life, and no adult, educator, assistant principal, paraprofessional, school nurse, counselor, or principal, had the wisdom or a conscience to refer Dick to a mental health professional, not even a referral to a primary care physician. I believe most school districts have a school psychologist available; however, no school psychologist ever evaluated Dick. I have to say that clearly this particular school district personnel in this high school who oversaw Dick's welfare during the school day allowed him to go further into perdition. Those individuals that are called "professionals" failed Dick, me, Dick's family, a community, and an entire society. They breached their duties; they failed in their professions.

None of the individuals who were aware of Dick's scholastic failures (and many in administration, or all!), mental health issues, and dangerous resolutions will admit to any knowledge (and subsequently, their lack of action which as personnel in the school district was required of them) of the various red flags Dick continued to exhibit his sophomore year of high school.

Unfortunately, none of the many individuals I speak of was held accountable. Not only was that horrendous mistake made within the school district and the local courts, neither have any one of them (all who in their sworn positions should live with plain humanity, decency, responsibility, integrity to protect a student) admitted they were plain wrong. They all erred detrimentally. I wonder if it's difficult for any of them to carry on in an existence of realizing they failed and never admitted so. In my opinion, those exhibited behaviors are not warranting emulation.

It's probable some of the school administration and the large personnel had their own children who were currently watching their ways and learned from their ways. Children listen intently even if they don't act like they're paying heed to your words and actions. Dishonesty and immorality serve no one, especially the innocent child needing leadership from their parents.

It's very clear that all the people who Dick came into contact with on a daily basis deliberately ignored all the red flags he continually exhibited for many months, many years. These were no doubt red (scarlet) flags.

> And out came another horse, bright red; its rider was permitted to take peace from the earth, so that people would slaughter one another, and he was given a great sword. (Revelation 6:4)

Dick must have felt unloved, uncared for. Nobody cared what he did, how he behaved, how rebellious he was, or how he spoke to others in the classrooms. Nothing was forbidden in Dick's world. For what appears to be many reasons (there are surely as many reasons as there are the number of his onlookers), all in his presence left him to his own adolescent devices. It's quite probable he began to feel like no one cared as no one took their roles seriously enough to properly parent, properly mentor and carry out responsibilities appropriately to correct him, evaluate him, refer him. He was invisible, he thought. So many condoned his ways and promoted his ideals of being invincible.

How much did he offer to see her breasts? Oh yes, five dollars.

The (ignored, unassessed, unevaluated progressive psychosis) mental deterioration that was clearly observed on his papers, typed out on his academic assignments, seen in the drawings of dark art outlined on his arms, and the filth that spewed out of his mouth conveyed an illness that *was not* hidden from anyone. This outright continual displaying of symptoms signifying a mental illness was transparent and surely diagnosable and highly treatable. Anyone can see that all the *red (scarlet) flags* were unequivocally *unheeded*. I am sure there are many more symptoms that went unreported for various reasons.

Dick did not have to suffer so much, and he absolutely should have had supervision at all times. As you can see, he was *undeniably* transparent in every area of his life. He was crying for help. He could not have conveyed any more loudly his cries. His pleas were ignored and swept under a thick rug, and he was allowed by many to take me down into his world of hell. Those around him in various familial and educational positions, who had authority and an obligation to oversee his welfare, left Dick to explore his fantasies and carry them out as if he was invisible and invincible.

Parents and teachers, if you ignore someone long enough as they are crying for help, they eventually will get to a point where they realize that, in fact, "no one around me cares about me." Your lack of interest in a child will fuel their pain.

There should have been *no victim*! If those people who surrounded him every day (family, friends, neighbors, and the large high school staff and the personnel of all educational levels and levels of *immunity*), having a moral obligation and a duty, a grave responsibility to all humanity, would have taken their roles seriously (dutifully), they would have gotten Dick the help he was needing and crying out for. So many individuals shirked their duties and were greatly mistaken in not reporting such startling information to the proper authorities.

Sixteen months after Dick's completion of and handing in of his assignment titled "New Year's Resolutions," he and his friend of eight years, Pat, scouted the neighborhood. Joyriding, they confessed to authorities. They began dodging other vehicles and people in the area, waiting for those perfect undetected moments to hit me with the truck, kill me, and rape my corpse.

This tragic attack could have been and should have been prevented by the people who were obviously in the know of the *red (scarlet) flags*. The information Dick divulged to so many in so many ways through his daily living was rejected and refused to be heard by so many, to be taken seriously enough to prevent a horrible tragedy.

All individuals overseeing and/or in the company of Dick should have been adamant about reporting to proper health-care evaluators, experts, and authorities the strange behaviors, the writings on his body, the filth that came out of his mouth loudly toward others in classes, the dark clothing of trench coats and the dark sunglasses which he was allowed to wear throughout the high school's hallways, the failing grades, the conversation with the counselor about a gun, the abnormal storing of urine in his home, the need to sleep at his parents' feet, and the conversations with friends and other classmates in the high school conveying to them how he wanted to kill somebody and rob a bank. Definitely reportable information.

Apparently at this particular high school, students are allowed to wear vampire teeth. No supervision required. At the very least, someone in that school should have seen to it that Dick be evaluated by a school psychologist...or did that school not have one? Hmm.

The year was 2003. I am pretty certain that accredited schools are mandated to have a school psychologist available, if only for emergency situations.

For whatever reason(s), the encounters individuals had with Dick were covered up, their inactions leading to an ugly tragedy. (I believe it's imperative to record in writing all conversations staff has with students.) The chicken scratch notes regarding Dick from the personnel at the school were all that was visible. An unprofessionally written several lines regarding Dick, maybe they weren't referring to Dick, maybe the chicken scratch adhesive note got attached to the wrong file. Detail and accuracy are important.

As you know by now, I haven't minced words at all. I have been hurt and disregarded, and I am very disappointed in these professionals and very concerned about all the students' well-being and how these students are being assessed and all whose welfare should be at the forefront of supposed school leaders agendas and goals—the "leaders" who are mandated to report concerns, behaviors that are strange/dangerous and possibly criminal.

Who literally broke into that secured typing room and removed the disc from the locked box it was contained in? Who erased that disc? This disc was Dick's disc by the way. Who replaced the disc into the box randomly out of the order it was originally filed in? These crimes of burglary, tampering, and destroying information, each commanded a thorough investigation. There are absolutely no answers; any manner of launching any level of an investigation was never begun. Denials, unknowns, pointing fingers toward others, no supposed "professional" admitted to anything. It's clear that no credibility, even accountability, exists in any employee who knew of the many incidences that were ongoing at this particular school. The failures were many and magnanimous; mandated reporting was obsolete. Regard for others? Nonexistent. Even an IT employee was involved in attempting to retrieve the information. Hmm?

Fact: a counselor or an assistant principal (there were three assistant principals at the time of this ongoing fatty, chaotic mess) attempted to obtain information from Dick to "possibly point her finger at him" (regarding the burglary, tampering). She stated to the police officer as reported that she asked Dick "indirectly," wondering if he would make a confession; he did not. That was it. Done. Shut. There never were official investigations conducted into the various crimes that were committed inside the high school.

A self-righteous, aloof, and very large group of employees from every facet a school employed should have been investigated by a *police department outside the district, an objective office that would investigate thoroughly and methodically.* All employees must be held to the standard they swear to uphold as a body of educators. In addition, complacent mindsets in government offices have led to the wrongful protection of those who should have been held responsible for what came to be, the maiming of an innocent victim, experiencing continually many losses because of their inaction and unrelenting secret keeping; banding together, they remained "one."

The many atrocities in this tragic event that unfolded over sixteen months were hidden deeply, entangled, and never were uncovered; it all remained and continues to remain "covered up."

I cannot, I will not lie to you and pretend that I have overcome all the obstacles thrown my way unauthorized by me, indirectly allowed by others.

I suffer.

PTSD, anxiety and depression, nightmares, and the random late-night occasional calling to the 911 center in the middle of the night out of ingrained fears are exhausting and have become a part of me.

The traumatic brain injury affecting much, especially my short-term memory, and creating an enormous impact on my executive functioning has made it very difficult for me to find suitable and maintain that employment.

The fatigue battled every day to stay in tune with everyday living, responsibilities, and normal practices is overwhelming and confusing. As most know, tens of PTSD symptoms can be very debilitating and are a constant interruption to paying attention, concentrating, tuning out the constant noises and distractions. This isn't something that a sufferer gets used to; *every day is a new day filled with erratic disturbances. Impairment in functioning rules my life.*

My brain is changed, my frontal lobe existing with many fewer cells—cells I can't have back. It takes great effort to concentrate, fatiguing quickly, frustration and sadness jump in. I am changed and will never be that unstoppable spitfire. I weep.

The former elegance in conversing and the mature filtering that once worked well, having always and carefully considered another's feelings, no longer works very well, and the most effort-filled discipline will not always prevail. The crying children, the whispering adults, and the constant movement of churchgoers who are thinking they cannot be noticed or perhaps don't care if they are noticed (and they don't recognize nor understand the disabilities I now am challenged with) are enough to make me vomit. This is a whole new realm for me; the Christian who taught CCD classes, babysat little ones, attended many Bible studies and church services, worked in an elementary school private tutoring and playing with the children on the playground, interacted and played four square—these loud ongoing symptoms of PTSD have turned my world upside down. It's an unnerving roller coaster, never anticipated way of living. The symptoms are unimaginable; it's a new way. All preventable.

An extremely healthy woman with independence and drive is changed, and not by her own accord. PTSD is a very misunderstood disability, and most laypersons do not take the time to study it and learn about its ramifications, so a sufferer quickly becomes an enigma to others. The sufferer victimized again and again and again. Isolated, desolate, stigmatized, and forgotten. Just because I look normal and appear healthy doesn't mean I haven't been changed—changed and challenged without authorization by me, which leads me in my life to being misunderstood, avoided, and ignored.

A very mentally ill sixteen-year-old sophomore was allowed to carry out his number one New Year's Resolution, and I will suffer daily in many ways until I no longer breathe.

Many moments I feel as if I am succumbing to this foreign existence; the anxiety and pains are staggering. The life left for me to breathe is debilitating and tiring.

I wish she would stop greeting me with "It's time to log roll." I roll my eyes and want to ask her if she has ever felt these pains and had to log roll. The term she always used had now become an acquaintance to me and an unwelcoming acquaintanceship I could do better without, I always thought! Hearing that term made me ache and most often brought on the feeling of vomiting. Those certain times of positioning my body to prepare to log roll off of the hospital bed meant great pain, a pain that would linger until I was able to take more medications and go to sleep. I don't want to feel this pain. I just want to close my eyes and make this all go away. I wanted the physical therapist to replace her favorite term with something that would greet me with a comfort. Log rolling is the most painful movement I have encountered in my life. To this day, that word makes me cringe. The term brings back the feeling of the pain in my body; the amazing body God gave me included with a memory.

I remind the staff at the hospital I would much rather lie in bed with a catheter. It's just way too soon to get up. How can all these fractures in my body ever hold me up? The four pelvic fractures would be of most concern. It's much less painful to keep the catheter in and allow me some time for the pain to ease before getting out of this bed to walk. Looking at the bedside commode made me sick to my stomach because I knew the familiar pain I would endure inching toward the commode to relieve myself.

Scripture commands me to not "hate." Most of my life I had refrained from even uttering that term in any context. I wanted to live by the Word of God; however, a lot of days I have murmured, "I hate what happened to me!" Can this pain eventually end my life? "I am asking you, God, to please help me live long enough to raise the son you gave me to raise and love, but if you do take me to your kingdom now, I would no longer hurt, but please let me live!" A constant battle of confusion always in my midst. Everything seems crooked, wayward, unstable, just pure chaotic.

Why does it hurt to breathe? You want me to cough really hard? It hurts so badly all over when you instruct me to do these things for you that you say will help me to recover. It doesn't make sense to me what you keep asking of me. I am really sick and tired of your demands.

I have heard that "pain is gain." People say that often to encourage others to exercise to extremes (enticing them to make them believe their hard work will pay off in the end, a reaching of their goals); it's worse before it gets better. That's not something I would place within my psyche when near death with my mind and body, fighting hard to fight off the demises of my new body and my new mind. If you have experienced a severe hardship in your life, you have come to the realization that this mantra of "pain is gain" *does not* fruitfully apply to most circumstances. When meeting new challenges, especially those that are unauthorized, clichés may come to mind, suggesting helpfulness but oftentimes a reminder that my path is not your path; therefore, your advice is definitely not useful.

A battle goes on—a battle to choose life to raise my son loaned to me by God; my son continues to deserve a good mother to love and continue to raise, guide, and direct him. I prayed to have a son, and I have much work to do so that I can follow through with my promises to God to raise my (his) son well.

This whirling of thoughts and chaos of living and dying and wondering and of much confusion needs to stop! But does this cruel, unasked-for attack upon my body and brain mean that I won't be on the ski hill with my son anymore? It's pretty evident that we won't be taking walks in the evening anytime in the near future, that's for sure.

As anticipated, the walks in the hospital were short. I was supported greatly by a wheeled walker. Not in a snobby manner, more so in a confident manner, I was proud that I was able to be off of the hospital bed and softly walking in the hallway. As time passed, the tennis balls on the bottom of the walker would require replacement as I definitely was in a mindset that I wanted to move and live.

Some days I feel I can do this, and other days I think that this just isn't going to work for me. If I can't walk up a couple of stairs, this evaluation board isn't going to allow me to go home. If I don't start hiding this anxiety and depression, this evaluation board isn't going to allow me to go home.

I hate taking all these Tylenol and Advil medicines, but it's hard to find relief. Walking, strengthening, riding my bike, it's not changing anything. I ache.

Summer is arriving, and the outside track of the hospital (the outside part of the roof of the hospital) is the place I am assigned to complete my physical therapy sessions. With the help of the wonderful nursing staff, I don my velvety blue workout outfit and wheeled to therapy. That area isn't just for physical therapy; it's where my priest friends and others would come to talk to me in the early evenings as I worked to progress in walking, sometimes just barely moving. I always loved seeing the clergy before I go to sleep. I felt so safe and secure when they came to pray with me. I still pray the prayer I was given sixteen years ago. God, in his faithfulness, provided his people to me to assist me in my healing. I may ache, but he is healing me.

Time passes…time passes so quickly for me.

Definitely not a superwoman, but I was at a point where I knew that I would do my best to stay alive in my body, in my mind, in my spirit, and in my soul. I had much to prove to myself and to Dick that I was not going to let his actions encourage me to succumb to his resolutions. I had to show him and myself that he would not kill my spirit and I will not give up on being a great mother to my son; I will fight hard. The decision was made to live. There can be no more vacillating, I chastised myself. Yes, there has been continual vacillation.

No, Dick and his associate, Pat, did not kill me as planned and hoped for on that beautiful Tuesday evening, May 27, 2003. I am alive, and I must move forward with this fight to do what God has given me to do on his earth. Maimed me? To a great extent. Created unending physical pain? Every waking moment. Created confusion? Yes, that too.

I must be the best mother I can be to God's son, the child he has loaned to me to guide, love, and guard.

"Go away!" "Stop telling me that I am repeating myself!" "There's no compassion here!"

In this instant, I knew I did not like this speech therapist. I never wanted to see her face again. I don't think I did see her again. "*People are telling me that you are repeating yourself.*" I don't know who she is talking about; no one has told me anything like that, and my people are honest people and they would tell me if they thought there was a problem…or would they? No, they wouldn't. They don't want me to have any more sadness, sorrow, and bad news. My people know that there's probably very little more bad news that I can healthily fully handle! What she was telling me was something I did not want to believe. (Sixteen years later, I weep. There are things I've lost that I never would have imagined losing. It's not that I had taken things for granted, but my memory served me very well in my life.) As I share this with you, my readers, I am getting hot and faint feeling. I am reliving being in the hospital; my back is in excruciating pain. I must stop writing tonight. I am sad, in pain, and I need to go lie down. I have an impeccable memory.

"Get out of here. I never want to see you again!"

"Who do you think you are? All dressed up and hair and makeup done to a tee. You think you are pretty special, don't you?"

Can't she use some encouraging or even some close-to-nice ways of revealing to me my newly arrived deficits!

It was determined that the frontal lobe of my brain was damaged during the attack, and as quick as a snap of the fingers, I have a severe short-term memory problem, which has proven thousands of times to be very problematic for me and all those around me. I volunteered very little about the actual brain damage; it's very difficult to admit that I have a damaged brain that does not function as it had for forty years prior. Stigmas are attached to those who have disabilities...you know that. Stigmas are attached to a lot of people...for many reasons—unauthorized reasons.

If I share that I have a brain injury, people will judge me, I will be "less than." People are mean and will make fun of me and talk about me behind my back. I wouldn't be considered "intelligent" anymore. There was so much transpiring all around me physically, mentally, emotionally, and spiritually. I feel like I was being pushed and pulled in many directions and was very overwhelmed with any interaction. This is very exhausting to me.

"Please don't leave me!" I was terrified of being left alone in that hospital. Even though I trusted God in whatever he decided about my life (well,

I proclaimed out loud that I did), I didn't want to be alone in that hospital. I didn't want to close my eyes. That would be closer to death, and I wouldn't live to see my son. I am petrified; I am feeling lost.

I was told my five brothers and sisters drove from out of state to comfort me. I don't remember them being with me. There was evidence people came to see me as they were bearing gifts. I remember seeing one lady named Mary, but they say there were hundreds of people stopping by to encourage me. I don't remember opening the cards, enjoying the gifts, or reading the words people shared with me to give me their love and support. Did any of that really happen? I don't know. You could tell me yes or you could tell me no. I have no memory of those twenty-four days in the hospital.

That Mary lady brought me an inspirational book. She had to leave as I became weary and faint. Anxiety and pain were never-ending. Mary's gesture was nice: sharing God's words with me, words that I believed in. His words that she *probably* shared with me were his words that he would never abandon me. I am just guessing as those particular scriptures would be relevant to the circumstances, right? God's word is relevant in all life; take the time to seek his face.

Mary is the only person I remember having contact with during my near-month long hospital visit.

I could be having a nightmare. Obviously, I am not at all certain of much right now. Seems the nightmares have hit me quickly. I can't say if this is a real event or a nightmare. It was as if someone appeared saying that my son had an accident on his trick bike and his head was being stitched up at a clinic. Have I recently denoted that I didn't want to be left alone in the hospital? I felt better if someone was near me. Staff is short. Perhaps many hospitals long for adequate staff. Now I just wanted to run out to be with my son. It's impossible. I can hardly remove myself from this hospital bed and much less walk and certainly cannot walk alone. None of this should even be happening. I am helpless, still. I am confined, and I am unable to help my fourteen-year-old son. I am angry. I am sad. I am exhausted, mad, and feeling imprisoned—imprisoned in every way imaginable because of some boy's resolve to kill me and rape me.

I say those words sixteen years later, and they don't even begin to sink in because I still can't believe that what happened to me actually did happen. It's very apparent to me and to everyone who associates with me that something tragic and life-changing truly did happen!

In that hospital bed, hearing the news about my son, I am scared and feeling like an inept mother. Of course, I am inept. I am hospitalized and unable to take care of my son.

I gave Dick's passenger a name at the beginning of this book. Whenever I picked up from where I left off in my writing, forgetting what I initially called him, he's now on his fourth name *because I can't remember what I named him to begin with*! Yes, traumatic brain injuries are debilitating in many ways. I just decided to write Pat's name down and then I won't waste my time looking back to the pages where his name was mentioned.

This is really hard.

I am feeling helpless and alone. Unbeknownst to me, the medication was helping relieve some pain but also affecting me in ways foreign to me. Between the medications and the newly arrived deficits stemming from the brain injury, I have no inkling who has been in and out of this hospital room, I have no awareness of anything, but by now it has been drilled into me that yes, indeed, my siblings were here with me from out of state, making sure that a thorough investigation was ongoing. They came to share last regards as they were informed that I may not survive these injuries. They are making sure I am receiving the best possible care available in this location. One hospital in the area, this is where I must stay for now.

I obviously cannot feel their support and encouragement, but they know that I appreciate all prayers. They have witnessed my spirit-filled life for forty years, as my entire life I have outwardly and unashamedly praised God and lived out loud that Jesus Christ is my Savior. They would keep me in their prayers.

As time moved forward and I was beginning to realize what had transpired, this was a time in my life I was thankful to know that people cared about me; people from the various circles in my life visited, prayed, brought me clothing, and some brought encouraging words and spiritual guidance. Sometimes I felt solace and hope. I was grateful for the visitors' care. The students at the elementary school I was employed at created cards, pictures, notes, and gifts. I was grateful to have had been in the students' lives for those five months; I know I made a difference. The students and I exchanged our knowledge and shared many moments of joy together. The more activity surrounding me, the more alive I knew I was. I knew that as I continued to believe and trust in Jesus, I was fulfilling a great purpose, pain or no pain.

I grinned. Those were five great months of tutoring students in math and in reading. It was a time of watching students overcome various obstacles in their classes and being with them after school to give them further assistance. We are all created differently; we each have our own gifts— all of our gifts are given to us by God. I was able to help them in a certain manner, and they will go on to assist others using the gifts God gave each of them. God's Word commands us to share with others the gifts he has blessed us with. Don't waste what he is blessing you with. We are to share, to be selfless and charitable.

I worked for a large school district, hundreds of staff in many departments, but no one affiliated with the school came to see me during this traumatic hospital stay. I wonder about that. No words of encouragement, no gratitude for how I once helped the students in the district. Of course, it doesn't make any difference other than the large notion that it became apparent that charity didn't exist in that realm, and that way of living isn't recognized as love by God. Trust in God, not in princes (human beings). I am blessed to have charity as I feel great happiness when I visit the imprisoned, help the poor, and love the voiceless. Thank you, God, that you made me who I am and help me in my desires to be like you, Jesus Christ. Amen.

Thank you, God, to nudge me to say that I am sorry when I error. Please forgive me when I am wrong. Make me more like you, O Lord.

I have always hoped that in some way, even in the smallest of ways, that when the students I made deliberate contact with remember me and in turn remember to be kind and charitable, generous, and selfless with all they shall meet. I always made my best efforts to shine Christ's light—my secret mission in the public-school district. I felt joy-filled and successful in the responsibilities I was assigned to complete. Those students made me want to do all I could to give them confidence, joy, and the assurance that I was there to help them grow, to soar, to learn, to be their best, and face challenges of struggling to read and complete math problems. I believed in them and they felt it.

As a middle-school graduate, my son should have been experiencing the feeling of immense joys, accomplishments, bouts of laughter, and suspected guffaws! Those gifts were stolen from my son; my son instead was filled with fright, shock, and hurt.

My son graduated from middle school.

My vision was not taken from me in the attempted deliberate homicide crime, so I was able to watch a DVD that was made of the graduation ceremony. He looks sad. He looks like he just lost his best friend. No, he didn't lose his best friend; he lost the "person" in his mother that he came to know very well in the past fourteen years. That mom of those fourteen years was gone. That active, fun, vibrant, quick, cheerful, easygoing, and extroverted mother was taken from her son on May 27, 2003, at 8:46 p.m., just before dusk.

This is not excusable, so many things wrongly taken. Will I see that unmistakable twinkle in his eye? Will I?

What he was now attempting to process was the stark removal of his "mom" who was left for dead on that beautiful dusk-approaching day—his mom who was found to be broken physically, emotionally, socially, and mentally and, frighteningly, spiritually.

He didn't know this for certain then, but he would soon know and watch and find out that there would be no more skiing together, no more jogging, no more fun gatherings with friends, no more hardy laughter, and all communication would be a new endeavor filled with my forgetfulness, impatience, and agitation. My existence was surely crowded by confusion. Life was changed. He would now have to adjust, immediately become adult, and maturely adapt to the conversations whose topics that were duplicated often became a mess of confusion. Fatty chaos is how I label the immense changes we must adjust to to have even a short conversation. Why? Because I can't remember. The conversations I have with others are filled with me demanding they repeat and most likely request that they reorganize their statements to help me to understand and grasp what is being discussed. It's a merry-go-round, and it's never a pleasant life. Let me keep this simple. It's a lot of work to converse with me. My short-term memory is destroyed. You may think that it does not cause much of an issue. It's dangerous to relationships, it's frustrating to all in the conversation, and it's stigmatizing and marginalizing. It takes a lot of work to have a conversation with me and enjoy it. Turns out none of us enjoy it. It's a lot of work, followed by tears (like right now!). It's easier to be alone and not try to participate in all activities and conversations and reunions I once lived with in ease.

I am one that has never resided on easy street. This street is even more difficult to navigate than the last street I strode. It's unbelievable sometimes how much can erode so quickly. I still do my best with the days that God gives me.

For many reasons, grateful for times past, it's okay, all seasons garner a purpose. At this time, that particular season was for an unidentifiable purpose. But goodness, why in the easiest of conversing with others my efforts become so exhausting, conversing with others will become a less-than-desirable event.

By the grace and mercy of a faithful loving God, I live to raise, guide, and continue to shower my son with time and great love. Changed and challenged, I did the best that I could do to meet his needs and wants. I loved him and he knew that. I have always had this notion that love prevails over everything else and fills another with greatness. Many things now were different, but the most important thing was that I was still there to be "his" mom albeit unfamiliar to each of us in many ways. He helped me learn to walk again; he manually moved my legs and arms, helping me to keep all things in motion, not solely physically. He helped me to dress and to go to the bathroom; it's obvious to you I'm certain that my son assisted me greatly in my recovery. I was feeling blessed. I had a son who cherished his mother and ungrudgingly supported her new life, encouraged her recovery, and gave her his time.

Limited in my activities, accepting the many changes and challenges, my desire to be even nearer to Jesus was real. I wouldn't be able to attend Mass. I knew God permitted Satan to interrupt my joy, but Satan would not interrupt my love for Jesus Christ. God controlled my being. Satan's intrusion was insignificant. Satan did not steal my joy and did not in any way distract me from the love God has for me and my love for God. The Word of God was with me every move I made, my Bible in my arms, keeping the words God inspired as close to me as possible—my daily bread.

My soon-to-be high school freshman became a caretaker to me with the interruption of riding his bike to the clinic to have his stitches removed from the back of his head. He would soon return and be by side. Suffice it to say that my son was an amazing companion. He persevered and his love and support gave me much hope and a desire to persevere myself. His motivation encouraged me to work hard to become more mobile each day, to have positivity and continued closeness with Jesus Christ. His presence gave me security, but I wanted him to enjoy his friends. I worked very hard to continue to recover and God sustained me.

Hospital stays don't necessarily all have negative connotations. A hospital stay can be viewed as a compassionate, safe environment for peace and recovery in a secure environment.

The most special of times in hospital for me was the impending arrival of my son and his dad to visit with me, share their days with me, and encourage me to play Scrabble with them. (To this day, we all play Scrabble together; much bonding and love occurred in the hospital on those Scrabble-filled nights.) I knew then that I would get very tired and be able to go to sleep and forget for a bit the pains. Every evening my son came to see me and that was the highlight of my days. Scrabble was "our" game. The hardest moments were when I realized it was just about time for them to go home; it was getting late. Precious moments of prayer. Thank you, God, that I get to play Scrabble again today with those I hold closest to my heart.

Have you ever been introduced to the reality that "as high as you go is as low you will also go"? Lots of ups and downs.

Some recoveries can be very unpredictable wherein the damages are not recoverable. The brain injury united with PTSD turned into quite a large number of losses. The former brain was an unstoppable performer that God had given to me on time, predictable, sharp, driven, attentive. I had the "go-to" memory! I still have long-term memory, and I will say that Satan did not win. My new life of figuring things out, completing tasks, and relating is much more difficult but not always impossible. I do and will continue to prevail by accepting and embracing this "me" I am just for today.

The reality became embedded somewhere deep that the "mom" who was left behind on that beautiful dusk-approaching day was found to be broken physically, socially, emotionally, and mentally. There is no more skiing, no more jogging, no more fun gatherings with friends, and no more hardy laughter.

Life is very different for all of us. Many losses are continually being recognized and missed.

This recreated brain, an unauthorized animalistic manipulation by a sophomore in high school, is unable to concentrate, is constantly distracted and agitated by noise, vigilant to and extremely terrified by unexpected announcements and movements and is now greatly lacking the ability to organize and complete sequencing as it once performed so easily. Plagued by short-term memory ailments, this new way of living has made job performance quite difficult. PTSD has many, many symptoms. They appear unannounced, and randomly, they, too, were unauthorized to be a part of me.

This novel brain activity is a very strange and oftentimes, a discouraging adjustment. The physical damage to my brain in addition to post-traumatic stress disorder is deemed a combination of complexity and difficulties in successful treatment. Flailing, floundering, wondering, and wandering—not comforting, nor experiencing secure feelings in this newly arranged body and mind.

What would be enjoyed as a normal enticing family gathering for my siblings for me is an overwhelming agitating ensemble of loud noise. My associations with them and most others are few and far between. I seek peace at all costs. I require a great deal of quiet to participate healthfully in this life. I am alive.

I am learning about what is required for me to maintain peace. Acceptance and understanding are paramount to the gaining of peace, and realization of changes is required every waking moment.

I have read many a story of tragedy and transformation, such as stories of heartache and pain wherein severe lasting damage has been done, leaving the individual unstoppable suffering, and then miraculously has been able to turn all the negativity into something amazing and positive. I will admit and you have already been able to decipher that my journey has definitely not turned into a "happy ever after." God's Word says he will be using this tragedy for my good or the good of others or for the good of "something," but at this time, sixteen years later, I am not ashamed, embarrassed, or feeling "less than" to say that I am in agitation and many a time, living in confusion. I have tried to hide the loud turmoil, the sadness, the pains, the uncertainties, the confusion, and the personality changes. I do not hide them any longer. I am who I have been changed into. I agree with and accept this newness. Did good arise from the ashes? I am tired. The mental fatigue and the continual physical pains add to my being of continually living tired and weary. The fatigue of the combined unasked for repercussions of the crime hold and load upon me a burden that is hard and sometimes feels too heavy to carry. At times, trying to sleep to avoid this all is my go-to. No, I don't want to sleep my time away, but sometimes I need some relief, and sometimes being asleep is a saving respite.

An elementary cube pattern is not a puzzle I can complete. With damage to the frontal lobe which is responsible for executive (higher) functioning, along with other responsibilities, I am unable to solve this elementary puzzle. It's difficult to iterate to you, but it's as if a wall stops any progress. A puzzle simple for most to unravel will never be simple for me and usually will remain unfinished. It's one feat of many which I am unable to complete. The beautiful God-given area of problem-solving was taken from me, unprovoked. I snicker and shake my head as I recall some cliché' used that goes like this: "Fake it and you'll make it." That notion just doesn't apply when functioning with a brain that is damaged, and there will be many things wherein I wouldn't be able to even pretend and/or look like I can "make it." I have always been honest, but this new brain is very humbling, and I am becoming more and more humility-filled by just admitting, "I don't understand this," "I can't finish this," "Can you show me…" It hasn't been easy to admit that this damaged lobe is not functioning up to its originally established ability. I am just beginning to embrace the realities and admitting to the lack of functions I am able to perform. Truly it's becoming easier to admit and it's unburdening me to open up and reveal that I can't do many things, I can't recall many things, I can't participate in many things. It's becoming easier to accept my impossibilities of functioning as I once did.

Yes, I am a believer, and I believe God heals in many different ways and not necessarily in the ways we beings may deem important or able to see.

Do you know how you work really hard to remember something and then the amazing light goes on? Unfortunately for me, that light doesn't appear most times. I have difficulties and live "out of sight, out of mind." For example, if I am not in contact with a person for a short while, that person does not enter my field. It would take something unusual or stark to remind me that that particular individual is known by me, and yes, I remember that person in my life. Maybe that was difficult to follow. Perhaps it wasn't clearly explained. Simply put, my brain is very limited and easily fatigued trying to solve issues in my life.

My first draft of pages shows me to type, *"Remember when I mentioned earlier suggested solutions to roadblocks?"* For example, some therapists will suggest to literally expose oneself to your fear that you want to overcome. Every damage is unique to the victim. No questions. Depending on where you receive your treatment for ailments, illnesses, etc., the favored treatment will vary because all providers have "their" beliefs in what it will exactly include to get optimal results for a recovery.

My recovery was in the hands of providers I didn't personally know. I was not well to even inquire of the providers' credentials, expertise, knowledge, and education. I would imagine it "was a given," that this hospital in this city was the one that would oversee my care with wisdom and knowledge. At that point, I knew I wanted to stay alive; that's all that went through my mind. I want to be able to raise my own son. This was heavy stuff, and my fight was to live so that I was able to be with my son! These words were my two thoughts, and those thoughts were all that was present to me. I have a duty to God and to my son. God gave me a specific unique child of his to watch over, love, and raise. I must live. Not only was my son gifted to me; he brought me immense joy, laughter, guffaws, and shared much wisdom and life with me.

My life and the success or demise of my recovery was in the hands of people I did not know, all were people I had never met. I was unable to sign any documents for treatment and surgery; the hospital personnel handled that. I was unable to acknowledge care required. I was a lifeless shell, and my destiny was in these strangers' hands.

The way this culture is moving, it wouldn't surprise me if patients began to make appoint-ments with surgeons for their potential care in their future. Maybe some people do just that. Make arrangements to meet a provider, develop a rapport, and feel secure if and when the time arrives you need their specific expertise. In today's culture, that provider may be on your speed dial.

We make every attempt to develop a rapport with many others in our lives to help us feel secure. I don't think my words of curiosity are too far off. A reminder to myself and to my readers: we are in very little control of much in our lives.

Time is passing.

The bright lights, the long lines of visitors (or interested strangers and spectators), the continual bleeps and sounds of gargantuan machinery nestled between the wall and my hospital bed, the constant demands by others for me to "log roll," "get up and walk," the continual activities of life in the hallways of a busy hospital literally made me sick to my stomach. Unfortunately, with this ongoing chaos, my brain was never given a chance to rest. My belief that I should have been given the essential time and space for quiet for optimal healing remains. I have learned much, and placing myself in a busy world in the effort to succeed and compete and grow and live big is not what will help me live healthily in mind, body, soul, and spirit. A big lesson learned—learned on my own. Living for years and realizing that what is expected of most and desired by most is not necessarily right for me. Simply put, those ways do not and will not work for my benefit. Misinformation in my many medical circles to stay abreast of as much as I could was something that became detrimental to my existence. Living as I was instructed to, left to my own devices, not expecting anything detrimental to continue on with my life the way I thought was just the norm, I became increasingly overwhelmed, fatigued, confused and eventually became a bed-ridden woman. Lack of information and years of misinformation were truly leading me rapidly to an early death.

Please don't think I am ungrateful. I am thankful for many things in my life. I just want people to do all that they can to get correct information or to remind onlookers, family, and friends to do all that they can to assist the sufferer by obtaining the correct information so that the victim can live her best life possible with the changes and challenges she is dealt. If you are an interested party to one experiencing difficulties, you will see to it that you are doing all you can to make things a little easier, a little clearer, or even just a miniscule more understandable to someone who is having a more difficult time than in times past. Don't leave a victim behind. Brain injuries are debilitating. If you have information that can help those who are disabled, be gracious in sharing.

I didn't know this then, but I do now. Sixteen years later, PTSD, combined with a traumatic brain injury, is a very difficult togetherness to successfully treat.

The providers had never met me previously. Obviously, they didn't know me (nor inquire information from those who did know me) nor how this brain injury was affecting me. In my own curiously evolving hindsight, it's evident there are many areas of my brain damage that were left unassessed. The brain damage was simply not addressed other than the fact that it was "established" I was having difficulty with my short-term memory. Providers didn't investigate, nor did they refer me to experts that would have knowledge to evaluate and treat the obvious manifestations of the brain injury. They were right now concerned with addressing all issues related to do whatever it would take to keep me alive. I understand and agree. Unfortunately, I never did receive specific care, necessary referrals, intricate diagnoses, or any subsequent treatments to help assist me to adjust and thrive in life with this new damage to this beautiful organ: my brain. Removing myself from chaotic-filled, terrible memory-laden streets, sounds, sights, and people, my peacefulness is evolving, and a healing is beginning. I am grateful to God.

It's recent that I can truly admit to experiencing the beginning of healings. Doors were opened wide and healing has begun. God's timing. I do not feel like I "lost" anything in the years I didn't notice I was healing. God had not abandoned me and was healing areas I wasn't aware of and God was preparing me for this present time of healing.

It has taken me sixteen years to call my brain "beautiful." I have come to embrace my brain and its newness and challenges, cherish it, care for it, love it, and most of all, to be extremely gentle and forgiving with and of its deficits.

This is sixteen years later. It's possible that helpful information would have brought much peace to my days much earlier had someone, one person, shared with me the truth and knowledge of my condition. I let that go. I am where I am supposed to be. This is a recognizable time for healing ordained by God.

It was critical to think about what it will take to save my life, but forward, what about my brain, it's life, and cognitive functioning? Isn't that organ, too, a very important part of me to treat? *Since the providers' focus was not on my brain, my focus was definitely not on my brain.* They and I did much disservice to me and my existence. My brain health was left up to me and this was a new area of navigation. Prospects of speech and occupational therapy were omitted when I signed the discharge papers and conditions of discharge. I have those documents. The only focus was my physical ability to navigate up a few stairs to get into the home and be able to use a walker inside the home.

Concussion—traumatic brain injury.

An astute friend of my late father called while I was hospitalized, states away. Remember I told you earlier that the news of this tragedy sounded all around the nation? He asked if I wanted to stay in Montana or come to Mayo for continued care. He had great belief to believe in the physicians at this world-renowned facility and would help me in any way he could. I didn't leave the state for medical care even though I too can attest to Mayo's integrity. I am thinking out loud, "Would my brain have received the adequate care and ongoing attention so that I would receive a more notable noticeable healing?" It's not mine to know!

It may seem like I jump around from one thought to a feeling to a question to an emotion. It's true, I do. I wouldn't know what the paragraph above is conveying to you, my short-term memory is quite nonexistent. I see the word "Mayo" just taking a quick peek.

I feel like you, my readers, have become my friends. You have taken your precious time to hear me, to be open to what I have to share with you. Thank you for giving me your time. The information in this book is real, it's important, and it's all true.

If you knew me even better, you would feel that my heart aches with you when you ache. My love and care for humanity, especially the hurting, lost, the poor, and the ailing is large. I cry when you hurt. I cry with you when you are sorrowful.

Wherever you are in your life, make certain that you are true to yourself and do what it takes to obtain the necessary information, referrals, and subsequent care to operate at your best. I didn't have answers. I didn't seek because no one made me aware of information that should have been available to me in my state of being. I made assumptions. I made the assumption that there was not a way for me to live peacefully, to thrive, even if it was an hour or two of the twenty-four hours of a day. No one came to me with advice to heal my brain, to share information of any kind; therefore, why would I think it was important to do otherwise? I didn't know that if I lived differently than pre-victimiza-tion, I would find peace. It was not brought up and I simply assumed the experts would have given me the necessary information to live in a more peace-ful state. They would have shared their knowledge and information with me. Or to see to it that my loved ones were informed of the information if I was unable to process the information available to me would be an expectation, not unusual or bur-densome, I don't think.

Family and friends, inquire much and often for your injured and sick loved ones. Be the ini-tiator in asking questions, demand answers, and don't stop asking, especially in the areas of health and injuries that are not often traveled. Persevere in your inquiries until you receive satisfactory answers and information that is helpful. Be specific in your questions. If a provider acts rushed, continue on to get the necessary information you need to make life peaceful and healthy for those you love. Your loved one does deserve the best health care, unrushed.

Do not rely on princes to advise you, to freely give you correct information. Ask, ask, and ask. Don't give in to lameness. You have a right to learn how best to help your loved one. Information is key. Correct, nonmisleading information is paramount to gaining health.

I tried to keep my brain active; that's what's promoted, proclaimed, and sworn by many to have success, joy, and appearing bright to others, right?

Keeping that brain active *all the time* is going to assure you of health, longevity in your memory, clarity. That's what "they" say, so most people will live as such. For some, possibly the aging who are experiencing difficulty, it's a win-win, *but not for me in my unique circumstances.*

Constant mind activity is not a precursor for the positive mental health for a victim of a traumatic brain injury suffering with PTSD. Constant busyness in mind and body is not a precursor for the calming mental health of a traumatic brain injury sufferer. I am here to attest to you that our brains require rest. Rest to heal. Rest to gain peace. Rest to rejuvenate. Rest to gain optimal mental health. Rest to be healthy in all relationships. Rest to reduce confusion and agitation. I only learned this truth of the benefits of rest recently. I had been living frantically and frenzied to keep awake as long as I could, taking in all kinds of information, to the point of feeling rummy and disoriented. I was not healing my brain living with the programs some suggest.

The culture today lives and (supposedly) thrives in a perpetual noisy environment, one of loudness, chatter, booming with busyness, activity after activity, membership to membership, social group to gym group. People believe they are thriving and living the good life, such as the nonstop workaholic behavior living frantically to one day be seen as a committed employee. As the family and health of all suffer, this is not of God. This is not how God wants us to exist in our lives. This was not his plan for us. This culture is not what God intended for us. Seek his voice, listen to him, and you can have those moments his creation experienced for a short period of time in that garden. It's in those moments you will begin to heal and heal in many ways you never expected. Be still; he is your healer. It's in peace that the Holy Spirit comes to us to guide us, to love us, to give us truth. Not only this. There's a tangible gift with his peace, genuine healing, and health.

I have, after sixteen years, wonderfully learned that it was imperative, following the initial strike of the forehead during the incident, my brain required rest and peace in its healing. A peace was mandatory for healing and living quietly. My beautiful brain was thrown several times around my skull, back and forth, back and forth, minimally at thirty miles per hour, cells damaged and deceased. A dark room of quiet for an extended period of time is what I needed. Not all providers practice alike. I hold no judgment. Seeking the "dark" never occurred in my thinking (and was never expertly advised nor suggested). Sometime ago, I was made aware of a victim suffering a TBI. The health-care facility prescribed this dark peace. I decided to enlist in their suggestions. I thank God that I was privy to that news report. It's been paramount to the beginning of my healing.

So it took me sixteen years to learn the truth. No time lost, I remind myself. I learned much about other things during that time, but from this day forward, I will remain grateful and practice what I have learned to be truth.

I paid daily for the unrest and restlessness; much has been unlocked. Here's the key: I am learning why I feel exhausted and agitated. I am aware now of how long I can challenge my brain in each twenty-four hours of a day. I know why I am the way I am. I know why I feel the way I do, why I do this one way and at other times a different way. I am beginning to truly accept and embrace my uniqueness. Sure, some may consider my uniqueness as a detriment to a fulfilling life, that I am living with less brainpower, so my life must not be as satisfactory as it once was. I am grateful that I have what I have. A part of my brain has died, and I must be gentle with the changes and embrace and cherish what I now have. It doesn't make me less than anyone who does not suffer brain damage. It makes me lovingly unique, and besides those facts, I don't want to be just like anyone else. I will not minimize my uniqueness. This life of mine is not a game; it's not a competition with you. It's my reality and I cherish the functioning of the brain that remains. I am a God-fearing woman with much love in her heart to share. I am blessed.

The "proper" healing whose directives sound very logical to me (of remaining in a peaceful dark place for some time) would not have brought back the attributes of the brain I once was so proud of, but the "proper" healing would have contributed in the assistance for me to be more at peace each day from an earlier beginning. I pretended for sixteen years I still had my God-given attributes of astuteness, organization, detail attention, problem-solving skills, and so many more. I lived fiercely physically and mentally *to try to make my brain work like it did years ago.* What I have learned is that I didn't fool anyone in trying to portray that I continued to have all the faculties God originally gifted to me, nor did I fool myself. It took a lot of effort and a lot of energy to pretend to be who I was not. Those many years of chaos and loudness and busyness did nothing to heal any part of my being. But I so wanted to be the woman God originally created me to be. It wasn't meant to be.

Hanging my hat on those admirable, intellectual, and energizing attributes regarded as strong work ethics has instantly disappeared. Like the flip of a switch, many of my talents were depleted and deleted because of a young man's uninterrupted morally reprehensible resolution. Because many people failed to intervene in a young man's deteriorating mental illness of psychosis, for many reasons I imagine, a lot of me has been taken away. I didn't want these injuries to be true. I wouldn't say I was prideful. I only wanted to be able to go back to a work environment displaying my former attributes, communicate equally and astutely with others, maintain a semblance in this existence, and feel fewer of these pains. I wanted life to be just as it was "back then," "before," pre-attempted deliberate homicide.

The effects of the adh aren't as loud, boisterous, and as misunderstood at this time; hence they no longer receive capitalization as I write about the crime.

Time passes.

I don't feel that way today. I have learned much, grown much, and continue to love much. I don't proclaim a bitterness. No matter the changes and challenges, I see and feel that God continues to bless me. He didn't abandon me, ever. I did learn that God's gifts to us may be deleted at some point, so share what you have, now. God did not gift you with talents to hold on to for yourself. Your gifts from God are meant to be shared.

Satan tempted Dick. I was for a long time saddened. His number 1 New Year's Resolution was successful.

Many, many people in a large community who knew Dick had sixteen months to interrupt that deteriorating psychosis which Dick suffered with loudly and outwardly, which was witnessed daily. *Sixteen months*.

Making a referral to the school district's psychologist would have been a very quick and a logical place to initiate an evaluation when behaviors and demeanors were witnessed—not a difficult feat to engage the professional necessary to initiate an evaluation.

I despise Satan and his attack on this vulnerable, neglected young child, who was already living a life filled with hardship, pain, and abandonment. The evil one attacks in vulnerable times. I do not despise Dick. I forgave Dick a long time ago, even before he ran me down to kill me and sexually assault my corpse. Hate never entered me.

I forgive the judge who I believed errored tragically in her ruling, and I forgive all the people who I believe had a responsibility to help Dick, those who had a duty to seek the absolute truth and come to accurate, final conclusions to all unanswered speculations regarding the crimes that occurred within the school prior to the attempted deliberate homicide.

I forgive all authorities for what I believe was work that was inconclusive and left as a heap of confusion for reasons I am not privy to.

My heart is unique. My heart loves the ones others will call unlovable.

Satan is Satan because he wanted to be like God. He was envious. Dick agreed to Satan's temptations with the help of Dick's mentors who literally abandoned him for months—actually, for years. Abandoned by so many in so many different areas of his life. Quite a few in fact.

Now that is a tragedy.

Dick's attempt on my life was made easy for him. Those in authority over him, who as paid employees were in real life agreeing to teach him, guide him, mentor him, direct him in the way he should go, but they lived as if Dick was invisible, believing he was invisible. No one cared about him. He was going to keep living like he was invisible so no one would find out that it was him who ran me over. He lived invisibly because that is how he was treated in his whole world.

Dick may have believed that since he thought he could control the weather, he then could quite possibly control quite a few other things, possibly other beings.

The "quite a few" are those who were obligated to raise him healthfully and pay attention to his daily welfare, and additionally, the others involved in his life were responsible to guide him and counsel him, encourage him, teach him and challenge him, compliment his best efforts and believe in him when he was struggling, introduce him to Jesus Christ, befriend him, spend quality time with him, hold him accountable, bless him, and nurture him. Most importantly, show him that he is loved, cared for, and supported in his work to do well. Just like all students, Dick needed to be shown that he was respected and important, a duty of his mentors.

Educators (I speak here of all educators including the administrative staff) are to inspire, develop a working relationship with the students, and if need be, their interested parents to learn about them. School personnel are not hired to *ignore students*. Bullies ignore; bullies hurt others and will act defensively. The bullied will react and live out loud and live their abandonment even louder by actions they believe can be invisible and hidden. Deliberate abandonment by our mentors creates an evil playing field, a boundaryless open field.

Dick tried for months and years to get any kind of attention from the school personnel. It never happened. He learned he had no control over his getting any attention of any kind from his educators, administration staff, or any personnel in any department. His life was emphatically devoid of support and all else which is required for growth, health, and well-being; his family severely neglected him, and the school district severely neglected him and operated as if Dick did not exist. This was taking a toll on Dick and encouraged him to run in another direction, to run toward or into something that he had control over, or believed he had control over, or the desired resolve that he would have control over me, well, my corpse, after the strike that is.

His family gave him no opportunities to receive mental health treatment; however, neither did his teachers, counselors, advisors, assistant principals, nor the principal who agreed to counsel Dick. Reports indicate, Mr. Less, the principal, never did give Dick guidance. Sad. This last sentence is possibly controversial as one report states Mr. Less did or may have met with Dick. Another report states Mr. Less (as the agreed-upon counselor) never did meet with Dick. I iterate this as it's imperative that all truths be shared in this book.

What is clear and evidential is that the consequences of not following up with a student involved in a dire academic situation tethered with evil desires written on an assignment sheet *are costly*. Sinful and costly.

When his "left unchecked" GPA finally plummeted to 0.83, it was decided, reports do not say by who, that maybe Dick should consider attending summer school. A letter was sent to his home, but the school received no response from a parental figure. That decision was soon struck out because then while moving forward, there was no follow-up by the school to the parents (culture calls it "phone tag," but this dire situation warranted a necessary connection, confirmation, a return receipt). So much information, misinformation, words, and crimes and so much more unimaginable or undisclosed antics dangled, and hung, which indicates irresponsibility and a lack of a concrete plan. I call this fatty chaos when everything is awry. Again, all involved allowed Dick's academics and deteriorating mental illness fall further into the darkness. It's really pretty evident that no one cared. I loudly announce that Dick was truly victimized in so many areas.

By the constant inactions of others to safeguard and redirect Dick, he was incessantly allowed and quietly encouraged to flounder. He wasn't made to be responsible to act and live in any other way (proper, with boundaries) than the way he was acting and had been living for months and years, for all to observe. There was absolutely no fee to watch this show ongoing every day for months. No one gave him any attention, no matter what he did. Good or bad, wrong or right, it didn't matter. It's quite apparent now he was going to try something that would really get the attention of others.

"Get my driver's license so I can do something that people will want to read about in the newspaper."

And people did read about his attempted deliberate homicide in the newspaper, all over the nation.

The passenger in Dick's Dodge Ram, Pat, did nothing to stop the impending and ultimately successful near-fatal strike upon me. My thoughts are "Why didn't this passenger yell to me to get out of the way?" I believe his loud deliberate absence of shouting out a warning or all inactions of many kinds contributes to the suffering that I live each and every day. The passenger, Dick's friend of eight years, is in no way an innocent bystander. A friend of eight years—that's a long, long time. That's many days of sharing confidences and truly getting to know each other quite well. His participation is criminal. He may say he was not involved, but the facts, his actions and inactions surely indicate he was more than a spectator.

He sat in that passenger seat the entire time Dick tried to hide the vehicle so others would not see him in his attempt to run me over. Together they sat in that vehicle, hiding in three different locations, avoiding other people in the area and also others' vehicles to finally strike me on the sidewalk. In my very own held opinion, one in which I never vacillate, Pat, the passenger, is guilty of being an accomplice to an attempted deliberate homicide. Sometimes, a lot of times, it's who you know that gets your name cleared from being held responsible for an act you fully participated in. His passenger committed a crime he was never held accountable for. Did someone do him a favor in getting him cleared? I have no clue. There are so many secrets involving this crime.

His mother was then, in 2003, and continues to be, in an administration office role in this school district.

I would say regardless of potential "favors," "unspoken expectations from associates," Pat wasn't encouraged by the adults in his circle to "do the right thing." He, too, decided not to admit wrong-doing and placed all the blame on Dick. Everyone placed all the blame on Dick. Pat, at sixteen years of age, was being taught how to get away with what you can.

This writing is truly a nonfiction work.

The passenger's professed *words* to the police, "*I didn't believe he was really going to do it,*" are not a defense, and this verbal profession is not a reason for him to be free from a charge of involvement in this felony. His words were enough of a testimony to be relieved of an arrest. I just will never agree with this passenger being cleared of any charges. Accountability once again dismissed.

This passenger, Pat, was named in the lawsuit that I filed against the school district. Clearly, he was a defendant; however, a judge overseeing this case determined that he didn't in any way participate nor commit a crime. He was dismissed from the lawsuit, and I was sued by this passenger and ordered to pay him one thousand dollars for his attorney fees, again, the judge ruling in favor of Pat, the passenger. I have to admit, this really makes me sick. Literally, this is sickening me even further. It's a tight-knit circle they are all a part of. All this really did happen.

The judge who dismissed my civil lawsuit against the school district obviously had some sort of, some level of a relationship with her daughter's educators, counselors, assistant principals, principal, and coaches at *the very same school* where all the responsible mentors failed Dick. Relationships that were possibly acquaintanceships, associations of sorts, possibly friendships.

There had to have been subjectivity in all the decisions, the rulings, the inconsistences, even if just "minutely" touching. There just had to have been. Regardless, with any level and sort of association with her academically successful daughter's mentors in the school, this judge should have known full well it was imperative she recuse herself from overseeing this lawsuit. She knew this school district staff, many of them. She and her husband had attended that same school some years prior and hold an allegiance to the school and the school district.

This ugly ordeal in its entirety was covered up successfully, that is, successfully to the human eye. All these people allowed Satan to guide them. Reminds me of the many plots I read many years ago in the book *This Present Darkness*. A darkness was present all right. It was in my world, and I could feel the evil evolving, just like Lucifer, like his evolving. Why do people have a difficult time in admitting being wrong? Why do people hide truths? Why do people assist in cover-ups? This obvious darkness that was looming for months and years was both hideous and heart-wrenching at the same time.

The teacher who received the typing assignment soon resigned from her position. The principal was cited for domestic abuse but was then set free from any charges. Could it be that this was the same judge who dismissed my civil lawsuit? The same judge who dismissed Mr. Less from my lawsuit? I don't have those answers. Just questioning things out loud is all I am doing. I could find the answers, but that's not how I want to spend my precious time. I assure you, it's a tight-knit group of people in that community. None of the many involved ever admitted that they failed Dick, but they did in fact fail Dick and many others. I would be included in the long list of people this tight-knit group of people failed.

As time passes, I look back at all the evidence I hold, and I realize that Dick wasn't the only one needing mental and spiritual health care. People who deny and lie are also in need of help. Spiritual guidance perhaps, mental health care perhaps.

Sadly, it turns out Dick's ancestors suffered mental health issues, paternally and maternally. I would think that a parent would be even more vigilant in assessing a child's behavior and seek health care when strange behaviors arise. Ignoring Dick's behaviors, actions, and words only caused detriment in society. Dick's parents lost their child to sixteen years of imprisonment, being raised by incarcerated offenders. These are lessons to pay attention to your child.

Upon reading the New Year's Resolution list, a school psychologist should have been contacted to assess Dick and review his family for mental health issues. *Bam.* It was that solvable.

It's apparent that had the school district evaluated and thoroughly assessed Dick when abnormal behaviors were screaming out loud in the midst of his failing grades, it would have been very clear he was suffering from debilitating effects of an illness. He should have been properly diagnosed and received treatment. This school district did much disservice to Dick, to his family, and to many victims.

The unawares and outright denial of the need for mental health care injured others.

Time has gone on, and I have removed myself from that dark environment, the neighborhoods bustling with reminders all day and all night, along with the physical presence of those people who contributed to the commission of this horrendous crime, by either actions or lack of actions—it all equated to a preventable crime. It became too difficult to continue to run into these people. It was too much for me to handle.

I have removed myself from the individuals who continue to rally around an administrator (Mr. Less, the principal), who took no responsibility for his inactions to help a suffering student, and those who continue to rally around him after being involved in a domestic situation that ironically was dismissed. I shake my head and remind myself that life is not fair. In my heart, I feel sad that none of them could muster up a scant amount of humility to admit even minutely that their omission of truth has caused a lot of harm. Not just harm to those of us who are innocent and victims to their ways, but harm to their own souls also. Pride, that ugly sin, has reared high for many years as you can now attest to as I've shared only truths.

I had to become removed from the thick of the dark environment to begin to initiate a state of peace and venture to the curious place in me to go back to read the police reports, the hundreds of pages of medical documents, the chicken scratch notes regarding Dick and a gun. The more I read the reports, newspapers, etc., the more I shake my head and thank the good Lord above that I am not one of them.

I continually thank the good Lord that I do not have to expose myself to those groups of people any longer. I was given the gift to leave that community, to remove myself freely and completely from the members of the community who I watched exalt themselves for many months and years. The self-exalting was ugly to watch. It was a poison I needed to be rescued from. There were things I could no longer watch.

It's been freeing to be away from all those people that I hold responsible for Dick's demise and my unending sufferings. They all stuck together; but winning, they did not. They lose in the lies. They lose in the cover-ups and the secrets being held. Deceivers never win.

I share my speculation:

Maybe those who were involved with the crimes within the school itself and possibly those who witnessed Dick's behaviors and words were concerned they would lose their (thought of) snug positions if they told the whole truths and admitted in front of the school district, school board, and judge that, yes, there obviously were concerns about Dick, many. The fact remains, no one cared at all about this student, not even enough to believe they were morally obligated to step in and step up and that it was their duty to get Dick evaluated, time was of the essence, and they failed. No one admits their failures. I don't understand.

I can tell you this, Dick was not a student that ran with the "in-crowd." It appears Dick was bullied (words thrown around the community at the time of the crime that it was possible, he may have been bullied), and he was obviously ignored and avoided by all school staff.

Someone, possibly several, made it possible to protect the school district in all ways. Fortunately for all the responsible parties, this whole situation could have turned out even more dangerous, involving many people. Instead it was just me; however, the ripple effect is long and tiring for many

It would have taken one short phone call to a mental health professional *from any one of the personnel at the high school* for Dick to have been kept in a safe place and quickly evaluated and taken to a facility to directly receive the treatment he required to be able to live in a community without hurting others. He should have been given an opportunity to get appropriate health care. He could have thrived in that high school.

Following the commission of the adh, the doctors' reports of the evaluation, assessments, and diagnoses of the deteriorating psychosis state this mental illness began long before he ran me over with his Dodge Ram. Dick was living out symptoms of his mental illness for a long time prior to committing an awful crime. Many months, possibly years.

As you can see by now, Dick's life on earth was filled with an ongoing desertion, and he had *no one* to help him navigate to a safe place. Dick's demise was fueled by those surrounding him because of their lack of care toward him and lack of any concern; his downward spiral hastened.

By no one in authority holding Dick accountable (disturbing behaviors, threatening New Year's Resolution list, a suspect in a burglary, theft, and destruction of property, intimidating Gothic dress, dangerous art drawings, crude, promiscuous talk, and more), Dick was supported and encouraged to keep doing what he wanted to do. Mentors and staff may not have shared an accolade with him, but even worse than withholding an encouraging word, their inactions continually encouraged Dick's abnormal behavior that directly or indirectly contributed to his failing grades in his "boring" classes. He had no drive to work at his studies. Well, what did it matter anyhow? Nobody cared that he was failing. Perhaps he asked himself, "Why not go further and harder and fail totally in my life? No consequences to my abhorrent behavior, no consequences to any direction I choose to go. No one cares anyway."

In essence, that very often wanton, unknown, unanticipated, unwarranted, and jeopardizing ripple effect from being ignored contributed to his disregard for human life and fueled his desire to have sex with my corpse.

Inaction proved to be a terrible thing.

I hold all the adults that had authority over Dick responsible. I wonder if any one of them visited Dick in prison. I wonder if anyone of them ever apologized to him for how they let him fall. My heart aches for Dick every day.

I will hold them all responsible in various ways, in various degrees. They all held different instruments in this orchestration of a near-fatal plot. As you can see by now, there were many plots, some verbal, some written, some possibly not even recognizable in this writing, but there are many plots.

I have been given the courage to unravel this messiness which could have and should have been assessed and corrected.

Did I tell you that I, too, am a sinner? This world is not easy for me, but I do admit my sinfulness. I have a spiritual director. I repent and joyfully confess my sins.

This tragedy wasn't specifically about lawlessness, injustice, unfairness, my sorrows and sufferings. Dick's incarceration with a deteriorating psychosis and the behaviors of adults involved and their decisions to respond in the way they did trickle down to children of adults who choose not to take responsibility and, in turn, teach children how to lie. People, this is ugly. This is pure evil. This is a covering up of many things which could and should have been revealed. It takes humility to stand up for what is right. The morally offensive cooperative is palpable to you, I am sure. What idols are for some will mean danger for another.

The many incongruencies, obscurities left dangling, unexplained and undefined reports are equal to a nonending and a most confusing entanglement.

School personnel are hired and paid to help a child learn, grow, use strategies to find meanings and answers. They are hired to encourage, help, and assist. Most often, those in education take pride in their obligations to be helpful and nurture the students. Being in the profession is not a time to feed their greed, protect their statuses, and climb the ladder at the school district.

I would believe that you agree that my removing myself was imperative for my sanity, and that, readers, is the absolute truth. I could no longer be exposed to the areas these people shopped, walked, and balked out loud in my presence. Leaving has given me an opportunity to open my eyes to all. Uncover some things and see truth. Besides, I don't want them to be at the forefront or the end of my days any longer.

You know how people look at you in judgment, ignore you, do all they can to avoid you or your smile. I always attempted to maintain civility with all people on earth. I have forgiven all who have harmed me, hurt me, and judged me and I have lived with love at all times wherever I have trod. I wasn't welcome any longer there. One can only handle so much heartache. I could handle no more.

I no longer had to run head-on into a school administrator of the school Dick attended, at my church, just to be ignored by her. It was a chilly place, that community, even in the churches.

Students emulate school staff. Children emulate parents.

Be watchful over your own behavior. You are closely watched.

a) I believe that there must be reform in this school district. I believe that when situations arise where answers are not given or found, an outside agency must be required to investigate. Investigate until the truth is known, known without a doubt. Proper authorities should be contacted, and all information must be written and recorded for accuracy.

b)   No stone should ever be left unturned again in this school district.

c)   Objective, unbiased agencies, based outside of the involved city, must be utilized for justice to prevail. A thorough justice-intact investigation cannot be founded when those investigating have ties to those being investigated. There must be impartiality at all levels.

I tell myself, "Ophelia, there's nothing back that way for you to see or know. That what was then has died. Embrace this present moment. It's all you have." It's hard not to wonder, I chide. I am human. I must do things on purpose, and putting the past back where it belongs sometimes takes much effort. I work hard on that which brings health and benefit, so these days if I find myself checking backward, I immediately correct my path. Straight ahead! Reminding myself quickly that there's nothing back there to grasp, I smile and embrace this teensy moment in time, embracing and supporting myself at difficult moments. Smiling that I made that moment a success to cherish and care for myself at this moment.

So I smile and feel at peace and embrace my very own "now." The efforts and successes to forgo "looking back" are huge accomplishments and vital to my health. These are not tiny feats in my day.

These are individual consequential successes guiding me to peace. I have come very far, and I have far to go. And of course, the time will come to leave this world, and then I will meet Jesus and be new again.

I can't remember what is typed on the page prior to this current page, but now, today, I will happily and gently turn back a page in this book and not be filled with a sorrow when recognizing I do lack abilities I once sharply held. I can turn the page slowly and gently and then I say, "Oh yes, that's what I wrote."

But, but, but…when I am forgetting something that I just heard about or saw or did, and I just can't pull it back to a place to remember, I am reminded of why I don't remember what I just heard, saw, or did, always reminded of the effects of the incident Dick wrote about, composed, and completed. (This is the offender's third name also, but I can smile. Please smile with me, and I remind myself that it's okay not to remember things and I make sure to cherish the brain's abilities and the healthy cells that remain.)

I had already made up my mind. "No" would be my answer to all questions looking for a "yes" to accurately diagnosing PTSD recently after the crime.

I wasn't going to admit I now had many difficulties. I said to myself that people would talk about my circumstances and I wouldn't be able to get the position I am vying for. I don't want anyone to know I have been changed, adversely affected resultant of the crime. If I do admit that I do experience this or that, won't that further my suffering, pave my way to be less than what I was, who I was? I can't comply. I must pretend all is the same. I am able to do what I always have done, get the positions that I want.

When I was working with him, I tried to cover up every issue that made my working difficult. I pretended I was not affected adversely in any way, by anyone, including him, while I worked with him. The truth of the matter is that I was affected by noise, background music, telephones ringing, people dropping in the office. It's hard to concentrate since the incident, and I am easily distracted, causing inability to get my tasks completed, increasing my irritability. We didn't discuss the ramifications of the incident. We minded our own business, we did what we could to take care of our clients, and he did a lot of work to salvage our relationship. I didn't fool him. He knew that I was trying in every way possible to pretend to act well, do well, and be well, asking him to place another buffer between our office walls. Yes, the softest of noises made my work difficult.

The truth of the matter is that I could feel many things beginning to slide. Managing my life came to be more difficult. I needed some assistance, expertise in guidance. I felt things beginning to deteriorate. It was important for me to begin to seek out suitable, competent providers who would help me to learn about the PTSD and help me minimize the symptoms of PTSD, anxiety, and depression. I sought out speech therapists to consult with to teach me strategies for the many TBI deficits and physical therapists to assist me in areas I knew I needed help to alleviate the pains throughout my body. I needed help navigating through this relentless pain that bombarded every space of my being continually.

The letter I wrote to my former employer was a letter of truth and a confession. My behaviors, demeanors, expressions on my face delineated a suffering woman who could not face the truths. I was a broken wounded vessel and it was time to admit that and confess my wrongdoings. The letter to my former employer was not an assignment to work toward healing initially. Looking back, it was part of my healing.

The Holy Spirit was nudging me ever so gently to examine my conscience, to look at the eleven years my employer generously employed me, to realize how my behavior and demeanors affected him. My apology was accepted.

After I began meeting with Christian highly-educated professionals regarding all my ailments, I soon realized why I had been doing what I had been doing, why I was living the way I was living (surviving). This information, wisdom, and knowledge were shared with me by experts who wanted to help me live a productive healthy life with what I have remaining to work with. I had lost friendships. I was constantly isolated and felt best when I was alone. I despised gatherings and frivolous, nonproductive, time-consuming visits. Because I suffer mental fatigue, my time of top performance in a day is short. I use that precious time with care. I learned why I was always startled by the slightest sounds and movements anywhere around me, why I didn't feel comfortable in a group setting, and why I was always extremely fatigued, weepy, sad, weary. Bed was my safe place. The providers God directed me to were blessings. They exuded compassion and a genuine desire to help me learn which tools would be of assistance in finding a peaceful way of living. Tackling symptoms with many strategies shared with me has been lifesaving, and of course, I acknowledge God's blessings.

Becoming ready to the seeking out of and being given the appropriate information needed is lifesaving.

My confession to my former employer was wrongly long-delayed because I never would admit that my behaviors, demeanors, and ways were effects from the attempted deliberate homicide injuries. I wasn't prepared to admit that I was even more flawed. I know we all have flaws, but I wasn't ready to admit my flaws were increased. I was experiencing new flaws. I feel very blessed that I have expert providers in several areas to help to work on becoming even more gentle and kind to myself in this newness and in the acceptance of who I am today.

This is the time that I have truly begun to realize I won't be that person sixteen years ago I felt comfortable with. She was a vibrant one. It took deep depression and immense anxiety to seek expert health care and receive the proper diagnoses and assistance to accept, embrace, and try to learn to live in peace with the many debilitating symptoms. It came the time to deny no longer that the outcome of the incident has changed me into a startled, lonely, and scared woman. Deep down I knew this was not the life God had for me. I have work to do to meet these challenges head-on.

The effects of the traumatic brain injury have impeded my short-term memory to a level of severity that is difficult to digest when trying to learn something new. I am not able to adjust as well and quickly to new endeavors, information, and statistics. Today I am learning strategies that will reduce frustrations from no longer having that one-time ability of impeccable memorizing and additional deficits and also willingly embracing the new beginnings at middle age. God bless you, Annette and Mara. You truly are God's angels. In the acceptance of, and in my grieving of the many losses, I am truly being renewed.

I have acquired much information from these experts. Did you know that damage to the frontal lobe is detrimental to maintaining relationships of all kinds? This damage I have affects how I make a decision and how those decisions aren't always positive. My language skills are affected, and those who know me from prior wonder how I have become at times rude and blunt in my words (filterless at times). Impulsivity causes great difficulty in my life and leads to regrets. Impatience and agitation are frequent (most times it's best for me to be alone). These are new traits which are not always completely manageable in a sufferer of a TBI and complicated further by PTSD. Today I am learning strategies to take frustrations away from not having that one-time ability of impeccable memorizing. Mental fatigue from efforts of finding the correct word and usage, deciphering information, and simply living actually is daunting. It's become a great deal of work. I require much self-care and a peaceful environment, and the people around me must have grace, compassion, and charity. I have to make very deliberate and important choices when determining who I will spend my precious time with. My attention to my behaviors is intense and requires ongoing scrutinizing. I require a peaceful environment that serves kindness for me to have peace. I require a noiseless atmosphere to preserve energy and strength and to embrace my fatigue. I require deliberate ongoing self-care without interruption from music, television, and chaos. It's not that I am one of high maintenance. I just fatigue less quickly when my environment is of solace. Being on constant guard and living highly vigilantly is an exhausting manner of living. These are just a few of the effects of the PTSD and the TBI; it's a confusing combination, not completely manageable on most days.

I have tried more than thirty employment positions in a variety of fields in the past three years; because of the continual symptoms that affect me from many ailments, I have not found a workplace I am able to be successful in. I continue to apply for positions, as I do continue to have hope. The vocational rehabilitation program I was involved with was not successful in assisting me to find suitable employment. I believe I will not be able to return to work.

Dr. Saams made several diagnoses regarding my TBI. Most notably revealed in my testing was the severe inability to organize; sequencing was a very difficult endeavor, and trying to place records and bills in date order for a personal injury case my employer was working on became a frustrating endeavor. It was heart-wrenching not to be able to succeed at tasks so elementary. My boss was very gracious toward me and always helped me along the way and never communicating to me that he was displeased with my performance. He knew I was capable of successfully completing my tasks; it would just take me longer than planned for. His quiet encouragement enabled me to feel capable and gave me strength to persevere and to be unashamed in asking for his help.

I don't maintain that much is lost with the changes and challenges endured moment by moment; it's just that my daily life is filled with unpredictability, startling moments, and what has become commonplace, setbacks for completing the everyday responsibilities. Having gained lifesaving, life-enriching information regarding all the whys, whats, and hows that fill my day, there is much more that makes sense to me. I am grateful for God's angels wanting to share information with me that would begin to bring to me a peace, the gentle beginning to the necessary quiet which is required for my existence.

The continual difficulties I share with you to complete projects, carry out my responsibilities and everyday tasks may sound elementary to most, but to me it's where I remain in my life; some things were just not becoming congruent for me to master. My deficits brought confusion and the feeling of a disorientation, and they do not adhere to rational boundaries. At times those deficits have proven to be detrimental in certain ways. The exchange and the firing of the transmitters in my lobe have been changed, depleted. Thanks be to God, it's becoming less challenging and frustrating to accept the realities and enjoy the nurturing of that which is changed. I am grossly incapable to perform how I once performed. I am pretty certain when there is such a shift, which is oftentimes subtle, I am now charitably afforded intentionally by myself, sometimes of grieving for my losses. The provider denotes that my diagnoses are complex and difficult to treat. Attempting to function as if I was the same woman who I was years ago became frenzied and exhausting and a realization I was lying to myself and to all others. Father God, please forgive me.

I am no longer "her," and after many years of pretentious living, she is being laid to rest.

With grace blanketed upon myself, my tear cloth is soft, and my tears are unashamedly flowing and wiped softly with my cloth. Maybe this time today I will let them flow a bit then softly pat my cheeks. My tears are not forcefully shaken off of my face, and I will not hide the flow as if I am in embarrassment or shame. My cloth will catch those tears with care. My cloth stays near me; it is gentle and soothing. God, too, will catch my tears. That brings me comfort. God has given me many emotions and I have begun to truly embrace them. I will no longer do all I can to hide what God has blessed me with. I will not hide who God is transforming me to be. This transformation is ordained by God, and I glorify him. He cherishes his beloved child and provides her with gifts and talents to share. She is generous and resolute in her desire to live in his image, to live in the image of Jesus Christ.

I now have learned to choose very carefully the times in which I will go to a store, attend Mass, or when I will walk my pups. It's important for me to be deliberate as to when specifically to embark on activities. Tailgaters terrify me, horn honkers take my breath away, loud mufflers immobilize me; I don't like to see what's behind me. "Will it strike me, will it push me, will it drag me underneath its carriage, or will this strike instantly kill me this time?"

I am no longer ashamed in telling anyone that I have forgotten to make my to-do list needed to keep me abreast of my responsibilities, my tasks. My lists to keep semblance and lessen distractions, realizing that forgetting to do something isn't always disastrous; however, paying attention to finishing a task is vital in some scenarios. I am learning some workable strategies and smiling with hope.

Importantly, I never forget that I have God who loves me. God's love sustains me today as I continue to greet the changes and challenges in accepting, working with, and genuinely loving my new "self." God's Word is not "out of sight, out of mind." I keep his inspired words nearby me at all times.

"I have no one to put me into the pool when, and the water was disturbed; and while I am still on the way, someone else gets there before me" (John 5:7). *I do believe the Word of God, God does not ration his gift of his Holy Spirit, I am thankful.*

I know what it's like to be shunned, to be walked away from, to be ignored and outrightly avoided. It stings. It's painful, and it's discouraging and detrimental to a suffering victim.

Please put on your kindness and live empathetically. Your deliberation may in fact save a victim from an impending suicide. Think outside yourself and remember that God did not place you here for yourself. He placed you here to give him glory and to share, to share your God-given gifts and talents, to visit the imprisoned (that doesn't mean visiting and caring *only* for those who are "physically incarcerated in a penitentiary"), the sorrowful, the lost, and the marginalized. Be aware of the meek who will not ask you for your help. Open up your eyes to God's children who need your time, your hug, who need you.

The lawsuit I filed with the state district court was dismissed; Dick's acts were not "foreseeable," says the judge. Montana Supreme Court upheld that decision. I believe that both courts ruled erroneously. Time and time again, I find myself reading over hundreds of pages of police reports, medical reports, the chicken scratch on a sticky note regarding a gun, the supposed "Pupil Action Report" the school created and maintained regarding Dick's behaviors. (This literally consisted of a few lines, which included abbreviations.) These rulings will forever baffle me. I will believe until my last breath that these rulings were extremely partial, magnanimously subjective; the rulings were made with astounding lack of truths and many inconsistencies, documented in the contents of this civil lawsuit. Dick was unfortunately never introduced to the special health care his ailments were ultimately requiring to successfully treat his *diagnosed* schizophrenia. Today he walks the streets of a large city in America, "the last best place." I don't know if he was treated for the illness while incarcerated or if he's currently being evaluated and receiving treatment since his release. I hope he will find a provider that will do all he/she can to help him to live an enriching, safe, peace-filled, and productive life. I hope Dick will be able to feel free one day. I hope he's meeting people in his new community that show him genuine care and sincere love with a welcoming hug. Frankly, he and his life are none of my business. I at times become curious is all. There are a lot of things in life, most actually, that are none of my business. In all sincerity, my prayer is for Dick's health in body, mind, soul, and spirit. Loving him does not require grace. Dick is a child of God who suffered extreme neglect and constant abandonment. I have surrendered much; I have prayed much for my well-being, health, and welfare in all areas. I have a confessor today that is filled with wisdom, knowledge, and a great desire to share his gifts with me. I am blessed. He knows me, he understands me, he respects me and accepts me. He knows what I need, and he is a much-needed guide and spiritual director. God has placed him in my life, and I am grateful for this gift. I seek out the goodness. It's paramount in our lives to find a spiritual director and let that gift from God be our guide as a servant of God.

I confided in a friend of many years. She was a friend I had on and off again as my inconsistencies caused by injuries and tandem repercussions were causing difficulties in maintaining a healthy friendship. I told her some time ago that I had been introduced to several health-care experts who were turning out to be quite beneficial to my health. She replied, "I knew for a long time that you needed some help." Those words were strong and crushing to my sensitive heart. The truth is, she was right. I was benefiting much from the providers I had recently become acquainted with. These were moments when I could practice scrutinizing thoroughly my responses. I learned why I acted and spoke the way I did, why I felt the way I did, and how to be gentle with myself and strategize moving forward. Before I move on, let me say something that makes all the difference in a providers' care of a patient: for a provider to be successful in treating you, you, the patient, must be ready to hear what the provider is saying. There came the optimal time, my blessing, that I was indeed ready to hear what was being said. I became ready to truly listen and extremely ready to practice new strategies, be open to learning more and open to the new ways of living. Some of the words I have shared are a summary of a provider's words to me in conversations. Becoming "ready" was the miracle to walk my path with a skip in my step, the increasing moments of peace, and the thoughts of potential exciting days ahead! I was beginning to feel the truth that I could become comfortable in this newness of ways. That's hope. Truths oftentimes can be painful, but there most often comes a time when a sufferer is prepared and ready to hear the truth and sincerely listen. This is the beautiful time when changes are welcomed, sought after, and fruit is in the air. Transformation in drive.

I don't hear from that friend anymore. Apparently, I had caused too much damage by the on-again, off-again components in the friendship for her to desire to invest any more time in our years' long friendship. I don't feel abandoned by her. I am now okay with her omitting me from her contacts.

What I do want to remind others about is that if you have a friend that suffers from disease, illness, and injuries and you want to maintain a friendship because that person is special in your life, do all you can to research all the symptoms afflicting your friend. If you want to save and nurture your friendship, become astute in their sufferings. Learn and live the truth.

The physical ailments, the many symptoms of anxiety, depression, the unrelenting nightmares, and the trickiest of all combinations to treat accurately and adequately is PTSD in combination with a traumatic brain injury. I began to feel the truth that I wasn't able to respond to treatment with any level of actual success, and the incoming information of this living reality was a cue to me to apply for Social Security disability. I would still try to work a couple to a few hours a day to keep myself involved in "life," being a part of a community, keeping my joints oiled, and doing all I can to be a productive member of society.

Sometime (recall that as I write this, it is over sixteen years beyond the crime I fell victim to) before I had gotten to the miraculous moment of "being ready," I had a harsh but realistic awakening in a position I was recently hired for. Prior to actually performing the assigned tasks, it appeared to me that it was simply inputting data, speaking to consumers on the phone and in person, completing mathematical equations for various verifications. I had done this before; however, the memory and sequencing deficits largely sabotaged the success I needed to retain this position I ardently worked hard to obtain. I have the experience necessary to succeed and I am very qualified. I have done this work before, almost identical work. Unable to efficiently sequence, my days were spent going around and around in circles, working the numbers out of order, trying to find the answers, checking and rechecking, constantly duplicating my work but unable to complete the equations, unable to conclude whether a consumer was eligible for services or not. This brain injury consists of blocking my memory, delays, and shutouts. Not able to remember which part of the equation I completed, what was left to do, my work became a frenzied work area with confusion, frustrations, and the proof that I was unable to perform the tasks assigned to me in this position. You would know that putting items in order are often simple tasks for most, but I am not "most," and these tasks were not simple to me. The woman assigned to train me escorted me to the back filing room where completed files were stored and sternly and loudly and at times with inaudible actions showed me just how far I "was behind!" Compared to the many other specialists completing the identical work, I was a long way behind. It was a heart-wrenching moment. I am highly educated, maintained high work ethics, punctual, experienced in many areas, and a fast learner, but I could not perform these tasks that appear so elementary on paper. With anger and disdain for chastisement, I wept and knew that if I didn't resign, I would be fired the next day. I can see why I was far behind, continually reviewing the document, around and around in circles for twenty minutes instead of the customary "few minutes" normally required to finish the review. My productivity was at a 2 on the continuum of 1 to 10. The constant distractions of chatter, gossip, and faultfinding, pressure of deadlines, criticisms and judgments heavily surrounded me, and I truly was unable to complete my work.

This governmental agency had no use for me. After applying for literally hundreds of jobs, unable to perform the jobs I was hired for, I was denied twice by Social Security, my providers continually suggesting and attesting to my disabilities. I was told to *"go find a simple job with less stress."* I have that denial letter that was sent to me. Their lack of obtaining complete records from providers does much injustice to many I am certain. This vulnerable writing of this book isn't about the harsh denials; it's about a transformation being made in spite of the moments, days, and years of injustices, unfairness, and the loud knowledge of the lack of follow-through lived and outrightly shown by many people, entire agencies, and several entities and its hired personnel. Many failures by those who were hired to serve the communities it represents, protect the citizens, follow-through, and do what is right linger in the clouds. We are to do what is right, no matter what transpires. It's truly difficult to iterate my disabilities onto a piece of paper. Most times the extent, the symptoms of the disabilities, are unexplainable.

Attempts at explanations quickly become filled with confusions, tears, and frankly charged with inabilities to clearly state what is felt, thought, and endured.

If you know of someone who exhibits my behaviors, my sensitivities, my personality traits, and you continue to desire a relationship with that person, please do some mandatory and adequate research to protect your friendship. Read and learn and do your best to understand what it is truly like to be a victim of such an array of ailments and tragedy. Slights of "Oh, I know how you feel because I have felt that way before too" are arbitrary, and highly likely words of untruths are condescending to a sufferer and detrimental to a friendship. If someone is important to you, you will care enough to learn how to relate to a sufferer. A relationship can be immediately changed when one of the individuals is subjected to harm and all the ramifications which will arise. If you love her and want her to be in your life, embrace the changes, inconsistencies, impulsivities, sadness, fears, memory issues, bluntness, untimely fatigue and agitation, and the repeating of herself. Realize that quiet atmospheres are heaven for a sufferer of this sort. Sufferers of this kind require gentleness and kindness. Sufferers as such do not make decisions that hurt you on purpose. Sufferers are struggling to just get through a day, most often. The sufferer does all that she can to help herself, but sometimes she will need your help of patience and understanding and the acceptance of where she is at, in this moment. She isn't being stubborn or rude; sometimes she is confused and overwhelmed, weary and fatigued.

Gentleness and kindness should be expected and easy for all in healthy relationships, but often today's culture does not promise nor promote the goodness everyone deserves to feel. If you care about someone who is hurting, struggling in their new being, their new existence, care enough to not leave them behind. Being left behind is a horrible existence. It is traumatic. When I am left alone to try to figure something out, I can come to a point of overwhelming anxiety rather quickly.

It's easiest to stay in my bedroom where I know I will find kindnesses to myself, by myself, and not fear another loss of a friendship when others find out I am not the same Ophelia. People tire quickly of my inability to manage the symptoms that bombard me simultaneously—abandonment.

It's not a secret that this journey of mine has proven to be complicated and oftentimes wearisome. Let me share some joy with you. Virtually, I am waving a white flag. I really am. I am learning much and feeling blessed to be able to continue my learning of what I must do to make the achievements to truly live my healthiest life possible. I am a woman who has survived many trials, and today, I really am doing more than simply surviving. I am striving to accept and embrace the knowledge and wisdom that has been shared kindly and selflessly with me.

I hurt at all times, but that hurt doesn't mean that I hold a grudge. I am not holding a grudge toward those who once were my friends or for those who didn't follow through on their words to help me. Truth be told, I don't have the ability to remember a lot, so it's probable I won't remember you hurt me yesterday. Besides all that emotional health talk, I forgive others easily.

My business is about me and my well-being in body, mind, soul, and spirit. My energy must be utilized for goodness and peace. No more running to escape, no more overeating to comfort the unknowns and confusing times. No more reading frenetically, trying to get in as much into my mind as possible to keep that brain active. Embraced now are quiet moments, listening to the rain drops, the ability to see the flowers and read God's Word with my pups who always love me, lying near my leg, the whinnying of the horses in the fields. This is the peace that stills the world which oftentimes interrupts my necessary peace.

To live healthily, my focus will no longer resound about how I believe that Dick and I were unnecessary victims of many others' inactions, impartialities, and subjectivities.

God's grace is sufficient. He holds the power to heal. God is who I run to. I have overcome many obstacles, and each new day has its own trials. With

God's grace and mercy, over time, having acknowl-
edged and accepted the horrific reality of how so
many *red (scarlet) flags* (were) *unheeded* by many
people, agencies, and entities, I continue to have
hope to continue to strive toward more healing in
body, mind, soul, and spirit.

God sent his angels to guide and teach me,
direct me to what is sufficient. His desire was to
soften my heart, relieve me of anger, and receive
the quiet. I have forgiven all who have contributed
to this tragedy. I forgive myself for being hard on
myself for so long. I take a deep breath and proclaim that God is good.

This compilation of ingenious feelings,
thoughts, and beliefs are strictly my own.

It would be unjust, selfish, and purely immoral
for me to withhold this perilous sequence of events.
I stand by truth, and I feel inclined to do what is
right.

This voluminous accounting is not in any fashion denoted for sympathy or assigning blame. This
relaying of information is my effort to persuade
parents, guardians, educators, and advisors *to heed*
the red flags earnestly in their individual capaci-
ties with their training and subsequently learned
responses. Heed the red flags attesting to their
responsibilities by responding in an obviate manner. For those of you reading this true story, if you,
too, endure a suffering, or find yourself "surviving"
(only), buoyancy is paramount to your health. Seek

to find the provider that lives true by their empathy and life-giving strategies. Ask the Holy Spirit for guidance and light. You will find that your provided angels will hold the line to the anchor that will help you continue to have a hope. It's highly likely he or she will have God as the captain of her ship, tandem to your ship.

You have certainly witnessed my feelings as many have been directly or indirectly denoted throughout this book, but there are several issues at hand that I feel very strongly about.

A *noble decision* for the state district court judge would have been to recuse herself as the judge assigned to the lawsuit I filed against the school district, subsequent to the student's attempt to take my life and rape my corpse. The defendants named in the lawsuit consisted of staff of the high school the judge's daughters were attending and the school the judge and her husband previously attended. For generations, the judge's family paid allegiance to this high school. These daughters were involved in sports and were obviously known by the educators and staff as excelling in academics in this Montana community. It cannot be disputed that the parents of these three daughters were, *at the very least*, acquaintances of the educators, administrators, and staff at this high school. There is an entanglement of various levels of associations there that should have been a stark reminder to this judge and to those who supervised her in her profession that *she had no business overseeing a lawsuit that involves her daughters' school administrators.* In absolutely no way could there have been any impartiality when a judge is in a positive constant connection with the school's educators and personnel of various departments that oversaw the education of her daughters. Judge Black should have recused herself, as there could be no objectivity *in any way.* Her remaining on the bench for this lawsuit was an emboldened straying from justice and of pride that continues to be a thorn in my side. We all have a Judas, and this person erred horrifically by remaining on that bench. I certainly wasn't the only individual this judge betrayed.

Addendum

Following are summaries of reports included in the main police report screaming of ambiguities. There has been no clarity and no answers throughout the events leading up to the attempted deliberate homicide. It's a chaotic, frenzied mess.

Pupil Action Report

Educators overseeing Dick deemed his New Year's Resolution assignment an *"inappropriate paper."* A counselor states he wasn't sure at that point if they realized the seriousness of the situation or the fact that the responsibility for the inappropriate list rests with Dick. Dick had been in gifted education in the past. He focuses his energy on subjects that interest him and lets the rest go. As a freshman, Dick was failing four subjects. The intervention at home would be that Dick won't be allowed to get his driver's license until he improves his academics (he obtained a DL in November, 2002). His GPA went from a 1.03 to a 0.83 his sophomore year. If Dick's behavior warrants, school personnel will "return to Dick's list."

Dick's Parents

"We're concerned about the list, but we don't feel they [the resolutions] accurately reflect Dick's thinking." They state they believe Dick created this resolution list to annoy the teacher and to be silly. They will monitor his behavior. They had one discussion with the principal regarding the courses and outlets for Dick's talents, possibly IT.

Psychiatrist's Diagnosis of Dick (Post Attempted Deliberate Homicide)

Dick's father reports a significant family history of turmoil and mental illness. Dick's paternal grandfather suffered from psychosis, received shock treatments, and began to molest a daughter, institutionalized in a state hospital, and received shock treatments. Dick's paternal aunt was diagnosed with paranoid schizophrenia as well as a great-aunt. Maternal grandfather of Dick was a manic depressive and was in an institution for a time. Dick's parents report that Dick never had a psychiatric evaluation at the high school but did have one in second grade. Dick's parents state to this psychiatrist that Dick has been "different" and "self-directed." Friends of Dick noticed a change in Dick two weeks prior to the crime. Dick spoke to his friends about a burned man, crimes he wanted to commit, floating faces above his bed with distorted figures, seeing things in the mirror. Dick described himself as "Gideon" but afraid of the dark. In second grade, he stated that "freedom was death." Dick's parents note that Dick claims to be able to control the weather with his special powers, saving urine in a bottle in his bedroom for over six months, and would sleep in his parents' room in a sleeping bag at the foot of their bed, claiming to see faces at his home. He named his mother Gypsy Whore and purchased vampire teeth. After the crime, Dick states he "tried to pass it off as if nothing had happened."

Diagnosis: deteriorating psychotic mental condition

Psychologist's Diagnosis of Dick

Significant markers for the presence of a psychotic disorder, most probable *schizophrenia*. The content of Dick's psychological functioning for over six months prior to this criminal incident had become increasingly atypical and pathoformic of mental illness. Indications from school records, parental interview, and social history revealed a pattern of disturbed behavior in the psychological and social domains *for several years prior* to the incident, suffering from a psychotic disorder of significant proportion which interfered with his judgment and decision-making ability.

Dodge RAM

Hardcore music, fantasy games, *Hustler* magazine (woman on fire), Killer Instinct, Final Fantasy

Student Information

On May 23, 2003, fourth period art class, Dick spoke about wanting to kill someone as a classmate sitting at the same table overheard him. Dick said, "Let's go rob a bank." The classmate replied, "No, you are crazy." Dick said, "Let's kill someone. We can get away with it." The classmate left the table.

Approximately eight hours later, Dick did try to kill someone. I am that "someone." Dick reported it made him feel "good and powerful." When Dick's truck hit me from behind, he proclaimed, "Wow, that was an adrenaline rush." He smiled. It's at this moment, Dick's friend Pat decided he wanted no part in this and pleaded to be taken home.

State district court judge *dismisses* the civil lawsuit which named the school district, select school personnel, and the offender's parents and Dick's passenger as defendants. I will summarize the words of the order:

- Defendants not obligated to protect filer because the incident took place after school hours and off school property.

- School officials believed offender appeared normal, one who knew the error of his ways.
- The "list" did not constitute an actionable threat.
- The district had no duty to protect filer from harm by offender.
- District is not liable under no duty in the absence of a special relationship of custody or control.
- There was no special relationship between passenger and the offender that would create such a duty.
- All defendants were affected by the dismissal.
- Judge did not specifically address the responsibilities of the offender's parents in the decision.

This decision was appealed and subsequently upheld by the Montana State Supreme Court.

I fought to win this lawsuit with specific goals to promote a solution to institute quality risk assessments and set programs in place. This was an effort to identify areas of training for administration, teachers, and staff and to adopt policies to safeguard the district's students and the community.

1. Get a drivers license, so I can do those horrible things people like to read about in the paper.

2. Kill the tooth fairy.

3. Stop screaming at my awnsering machine.

4. Get a job so I can afford ammo.

5. Improve typing grade.

6. Taste human flesh.

7. Make a movie about Hitler.

8. Find out what really happened in Roswell New Mexico.

9. Find out who really killed JFK and invite blood relatives to a BBQ.

10. Shoot some one on a caping trip and say it was an accident.

School resolutions.

Raise typing and english grades.

Sign up in a club.

Take as many math courses as possible.

Fewer absences.

Carry less books.

My Parting Words

Relying that sworn-to impartiality and objectivity would be displayed to see the benefits of the outcome of this suit was paramount for me to eagerly initiate and assist to institute the appropriate and necessary training of all personnel and updating and maintaining the proper policies to protect students and the community.

This was my goal, but the breaking of promises, the sworn oaths not heeded, lacking truth and honesty, *impeded my goals and deemed them largely impossible.* An intricately woven entanglement on various levels existed for years, webbings that hung heavily which were stained by various levels of associations, secretly undefined, spoken of widespread in the newspaper over the years, evident in websites and the boasting of connections seen in campaign support ads.

Relationships, undoubtedly friendships, but in the very least, *associations, associations which spoke volumes to all who read the local newspaper, but kept in darkness, secrets.*

The judges, principal, counselors, chairman, member of Chamber of Commerce and Leadership High School, realtor, assistant principals, coaches, administrative assistant, parents of students, all at the *very least, acquaintances*—I beg to differ with this operational low level of "association"; however, there's no reason for me to delve any deeper. What I have learned without effort has made my head spin and there's no reason for me to read onward about their levels of associations beyond acquaintanceships and the deep silence that was maintained. I've learned enough to see with my very own eyes on public paper, computer screens, campaign ads, and articles of many sorts that a deep darkness spews in this unfolding—a darkness that speaks volumes, indicating that none of them valued truth and justice. No truth or justice would be brought to light.

Through various newspapers I read that the *judge's* daughter(s) participated on a sports *team* with the *assistant principal's* daughter. These daughters *attended* the same high school (some in the *same grade*), an entity of the district, the high school led by the principal targeted in my lawsuit. The team also consisted of the daughter of a state supreme court *judge* who upheld the district court judge's ruling of the dismissal of my lawsuit. The *principal* loved and *coached* sports for many decades, boasting in the local newspaper of attending as many activities as possible. The ruling state district judge and at least one of the upholding state supreme court judges had a relationship as their daughters played sports together, at times, on the same team. That's the minimal relationship. That's common knowledge in the community. Those daughters were on the same team at some point. These are minimal relationships iterated in a local newspaper, my readers, minimal information shouting an inability for *this* judge to be objective, impartial, just.

These judges involved had a moral and an ethical obligation to recuse themselves from participating as judges in overseeing and ruling on this lawsuit as there is no way either one could have been objective.

The infamous counselor and principal at the high school I have referenced throughout this book were *mandatory* participants of a program in the community, which at one time was chaired by a member of the Chamber of Commerce, who is the husband of the ruling *judge*. He was the first chair-person of LHS. This program in which juniors in high school pay a fee and partake in informational sessions/shadowing to become "leaders" is named Leadership High School, an entity operated under the Chamber of Commerce. In order for a junior student to participate, the student must be nominated then authorized by the *counselor* to participate and then subsequently receive an approval by the *principal* to participate in the program operated conjointly by the chamber and the high school's counselor and principal. The one-time chair and an ongoing member of the Chamber of Commerce, at the time of this writing, is the *judge's* husband. Another loud association, an association which in no way allows a *judge* to be impartial. This is only information I ran across. These associations existed for years, my readers. The *passenger* in the vehicle that struck me, interestingly enough, was a son of a woman who held a position in the administration office in this same school district I filed suit against. The passenger was never charged. He graduated in the class with one of the ruling judge's daughters.

This has not been an entertaining puzzle to embark upon. This wasn't work to uncover all these close associations. All this information is public information and readily available to see in the local newspaper over many years and of course on your digital devices you hold readily in your hand.

This is a deep web, my readers, and if you've picked up this book, you too live for justice as I continue to do. I didn't receive justice. I had judges' rule who were closely and in many different ways and levels associated with defendants in my lawsuit. This is not pretty. This uncovering spews of deceit in various ways.

This is a web that has been tightly knitted over years and years, dripping darkly with secrets, quietly and secretly. Anyone interested enough in this darkness can delve even deeper to see the open evidence that this lawsuit ruling was ultimately tainted with unethical and immoral decisions by human beings in their immoral *refusal to rightly and honestly recuse themselves. These individuals chose to remain on the bench, to be the judges to dismiss and uphold the ruling. These individuals had no business overseeing this suit nor subsequently ruling on this suit.*

(This information is not fabricated. This information is broadcasted via the local newspaper in a city in Montana, on various websites, in police reports, and in the civil lawsuits.)

Good does arise from the ashes.

> And do not grieve the Holy Spirit of God, in whom you were sealed for the day of redemption. Let all bitterness and wrath and anger and clamor and slander be put away from you, with all malice, and be kind to one another, as God in Christ forgave you. (Ephesians 4:30–32)

> Therefore, be imitators of God, as beloved children. And walk in love as Christ Loved us and gave himself up for us, a fragrant offering and sacrifice to God. (Ephesians 5:1–2)

I forgive all individuals who have contributed in any way in the allowance of the commission of this tragedy. Dick, you were forgiven before you even ran me over and dragged me.

> As far as the east is from the west, so far does he remove our

transgressions from us. As a father pities his children, so the Lord pities those who fear him. (Psalm 103:12–13)

White flag flying.

About the Author

Ophelia is a graduate of a university exceling in her passions of sociology, criminal justice, and psychology. She is an avid reader who understands which subject matters are of importance today in our culture to be fervently read and subsequently embraced. She reminds us of the many important matters and behaviors that may seem inconsequential but that must be assessed. She authors this writing with unstoppable prayers, prayers for honesty, humility, and justice in this world. Ophelia is a sought-after listener and a survivor of perils who continues to chase after our Lord, basking in his peace and love.

9 781098 095192